GLUCOSE

REVOLUTION CODE

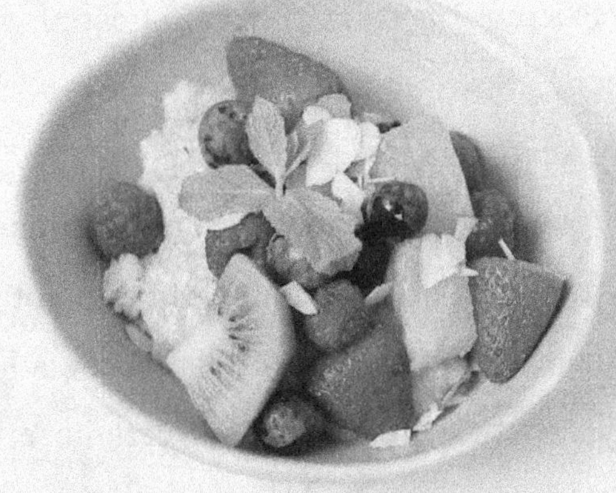

The ultimate life-changing guide for normalizing blood sugar

Dr. Simon S. Edwards

Copyright © 2023 by
Dr. Simon S. Edwards

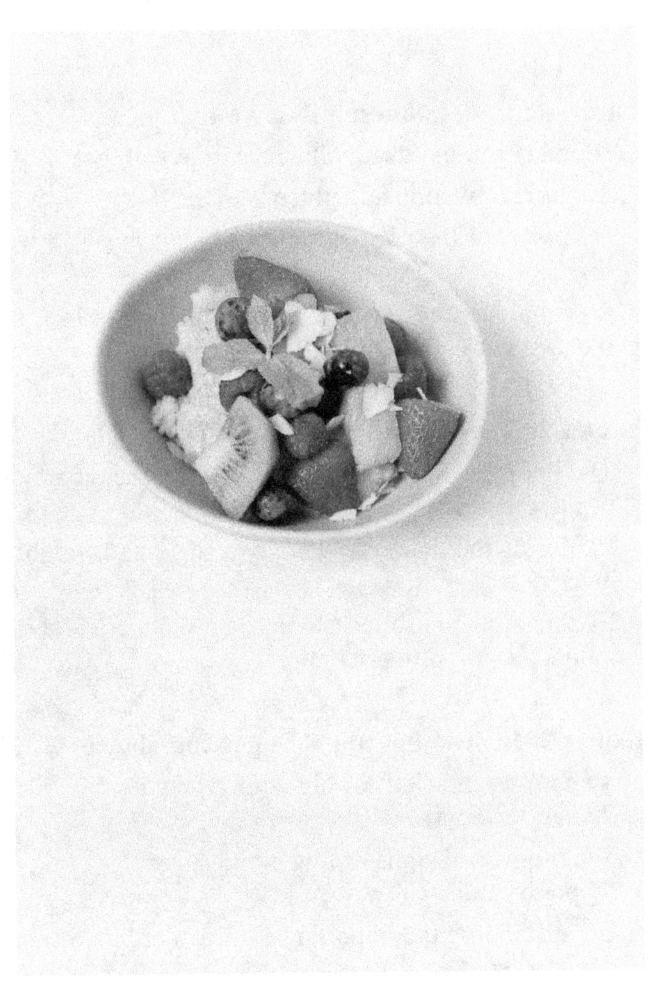

2| **Glucose Revolution Code**

Table Of Content

Introduction

Philip, a middle-aged man with a sweet tooth, found himself imprisoned in the grasp of uncontrolled sugar levels. He was fatigued, experienced mood swings, and needed sugary snacks all the time. Frustrated by the pattern, he stumbled across a book called "Glucose Revolution Code ," which purported to uncover the secrets of sugar level regulation.

As he went through its pages, Philip uncovered a treasure trove of information on nutrition, fitness, and mindful eating. The book presented him with a road map to a better lifestyle, emphasizing the necessity of balance and moderation. It went over how different foods affect blood sugar levels and how to make better nutritional choices.

Philip was inspired and eager to put his newfound knowledge into action. He said goodbye to sugary pleasures in favor of natural nutrition and frequent exercise. His sugar levels began to settle gradually. His tiredness subsided, and his spirits improved.

Philip's metamorphosis shocked not just him, but also his friends and family. His experience was a monument to the strength of knowledge and self-discipline. He resolved to tell his tale from that moment on, encouraging others to take charge of their health through the simple act of reading and studying.

In today's world, the prevalence of high blood sugar levels has reached alarming levels, with millions of people suffering from diseases such as diabetes and prediabetes. Maintaining normal blood sugar levels is crucial for general well-being since imbalances can lead to a variety of health concerns and a lower quality of life. Fortunately, there is an increasing emphasis on discovering effective remedies for this disease, and one such approach is the "Glucose Revolution Code ."

The Glucose Revolution Code is a holistic technique for stabilizing and managing blood sugar levels that involves dietary adjustments, physical activity, and lifestyle changes. It stresses eating balanced meals consisting of nutritious grains, lean proteins, and nutrient-dense greens while avoiding refined carbohydrates and processed foods. Regular exercise, including both aerobic and strength training, is a vital component of the Glucose Revolution Code . Additionally, stress management methods, appropriate sleep, and regular blood sugar testing are added to the program to ensure long-term success.

Individuals who apply the Glucose Revolution Code technique can acquire control of their blood sugar levels, lower the risk of consequences related to high blood sugar, and enhance their general health and well-being.

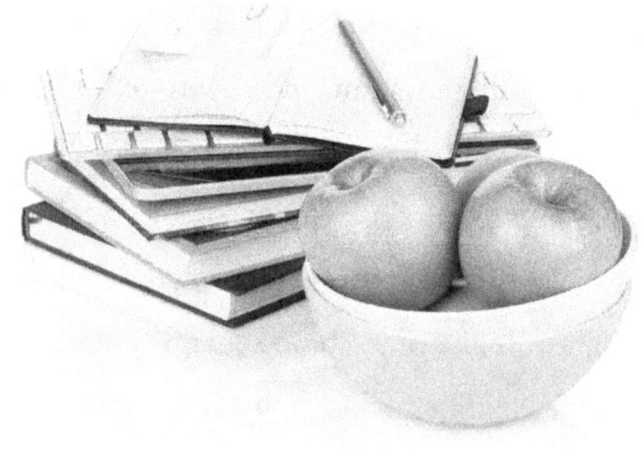

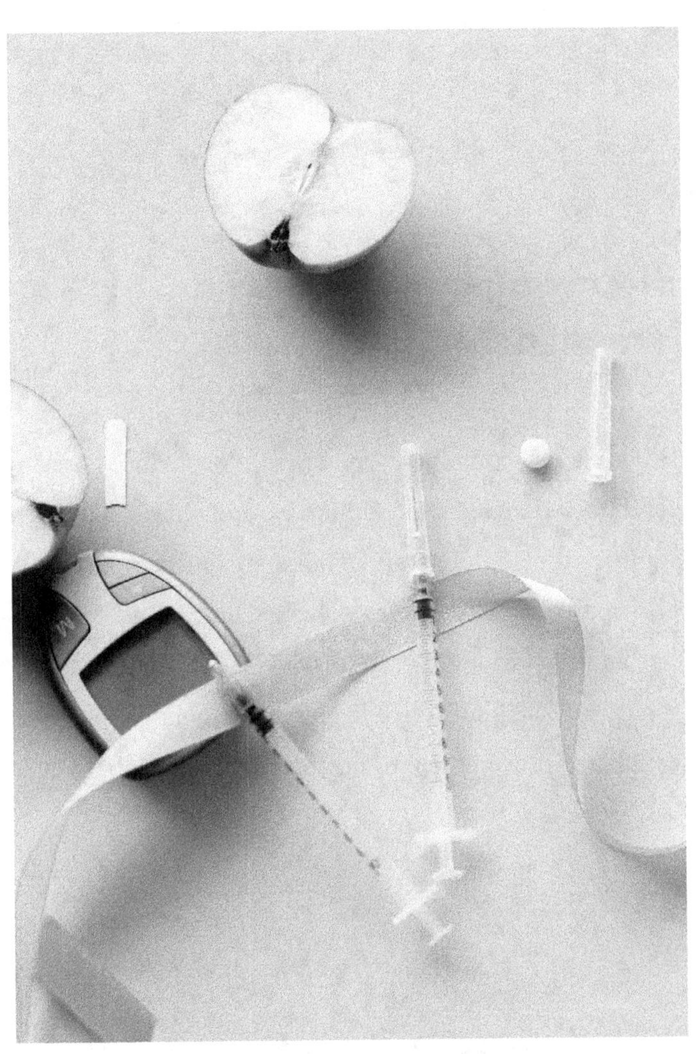

Chapter 1: Understanding Blood Sugar

Blood sugar and its significance in overall health

Blood sugar, commonly known as blood glucose, is an essential component of human physiology and plays a significant role in overall health and well-being. It is the principal source of energy for our cells and is essential for a range of biological tasks. Understanding blood sugar and its significance is crucial to maintaining good health and preventing chronic disorders like diabetes.

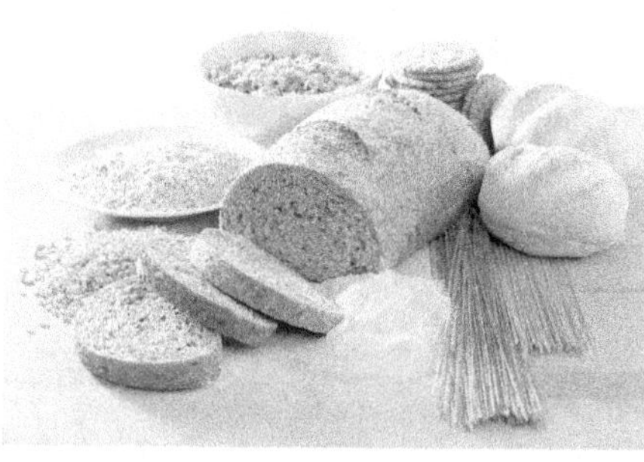

When we take carbohydrates, our bodies turn them into glucose, which enters the bloodstream. This prompts the pancreas to create insulin, a hormone that regulates blood sugar levels. Insulin serves as a "key," allowing glucose to enter cells and be used as energy. This system serves to keep blood sugar levels stable, ensuring that glucose is accessible to power the body's processes.

The relevance of blood sugar arises from its impact on numerous facets of human health. Proper blood sugar regulation is critical for energy metabolism because glucose provides the energy required for cellular processes, physical activity, and mental performance. Stable blood sugar levels enhance long-term energy, and increased cognitive function, and general vitality.

Furthermore, blood sugar regulation is intricately connected to weight control. Extra glucose is generally stored as fat when blood sugar levels are high, resulting in weight gain. Low blood sugar, on the other hand, can produce hunger and cravings, which can lead to overeating and weight gain. Individuals can promote good weight control and limit their risk of obesity-related disorders by sustaining stable blood sugar levels.

Blood sugar regulation is also vital in the prevention and management of chronic disorders such as diabetes. Diabetes is a metabolic disorder characterized by excessive blood sugar levels and the body's inability to appropriately handle insulin. Chronic high blood sugar levels can cause cardiovascular sickness, renal damage, nerve damage, and visual issues. Understanding and regulating blood sugar is therefore vital for avoiding and managing diabetes and its accompanying health consequences.

The role of insulin and glucose in the body

Insulin and glucose play key roles in our bodies.

Glucose is a form of sugar that comes from the food we eat, specifically carbohydrates. It is our cells' principal source of energy. When we eat, our bodies turn carbohydrates into glucose, which enters our circulation.

Insulin is a hormone generated by a specific organ known as the pancreas. It assists in the regulation of blood glucose levels. The pancreas manufactures insulin in the bloodstream when the level of glucose in our blood rises after a meal.
Insulin serves as a key, unlocking the doors of our cells and allowing glucose to enter. Glucose can be used for energy after it enters the cells. It's analogous to putting gas in a car so that it can run.

Insulin's job is to regulate the level of glucose in our blood within a healthy range. When there is an overabundance of glucose in our blood, insulin aids in its transit into our cells for storage or immediate energy consumption. This aids in restoring normal blood sugar levels.

If the level of glucose in our blood gets too low, insulin synthesis ceases and another hormone known as glucagon is released. Glucagon tells the liver to release stored glucose into the bloodstream, therefore boosting blood sugar levels.

In this way, insulin and glucose collaborate to keep our blood sugar levels in balance. They ensure that our cells have enough energy to perform properly and that our bodies can efficiently use and store glucose.

When the body does not create enough insulin or does not utilize insulin effectively, issues could emerge. This can result in hyperglycemia, or elevated blood sugar levels, which is a symptom of diabetes. If blood sugar levels are regularly high or low, it can lead to health concerns and consequences.

Overview of the normal range of blood sugar levels

The typical amount of glucose in the bloodstream is referred to as the normal range of blood sugar levels.

These ranges can vary substantially based on the precise criteria and units of measurement chosen.

The normal range of fasting blood sugar levels (taken after at least 8 hours without eating) for most healthy adults is 70 to 99 milligrams per deciliter (mg/dL) or 3.9 to 5.5 millimoles per liter (mmol/L). This range suggests that the body's blood sugar levels are stable and healthy.

Blood sugar levels can briefly rise after a meal. However, they should return to normal within a few hours. Blood sugar levels two hours after eating are normally less than 140 mg/dL (7.8 mmol/L). According to some guidelines, postprandial blood sugar levels should be fewer than 180 mg/dL (10 mmol/L).

It is crucial to note that blood sugar targets may differ for persons who have specific health issues, such as diabetes. Diabetes patients typically have precise goal ranges prescribed by their healthcare professional in order to effectively regulate their blood sugar.

Hypoglycemia occurs when blood sugar levels fall below the usual range. Hypoglycemia is characterized as blood sugar levels below 70 mg/dL (3.9 mmol/L). Symptoms include dizziness, shakiness, confusion, and sweating. Immediate therapy, such as ingesting glucose or a source of fast-acting carbohydrates, is crucial for restoring normal blood sugar levels.

Chronically high blood sugar levels, known as hyperglycemia, on the other hand, may be a symptom of underlying health conditions such as diabetes. When fasting blood sugar levels are persistently above 126 mg/dL (7.0 mmol/L) or random blood sugar readings above 200 mg/dL (11.1 mmol/L), hyperglycemia is frequently diagnosed. Prolonged hyperglycemia can create difficulties, hence managing blood sugar levels is vital for diabetics.

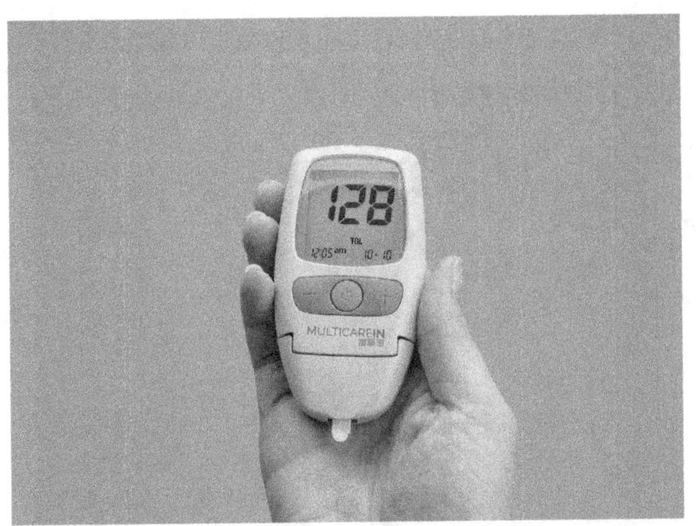

128
TDL
12:05 am   10-10
MULTICAREIN

Potential health risks associated with high or low blood sugar

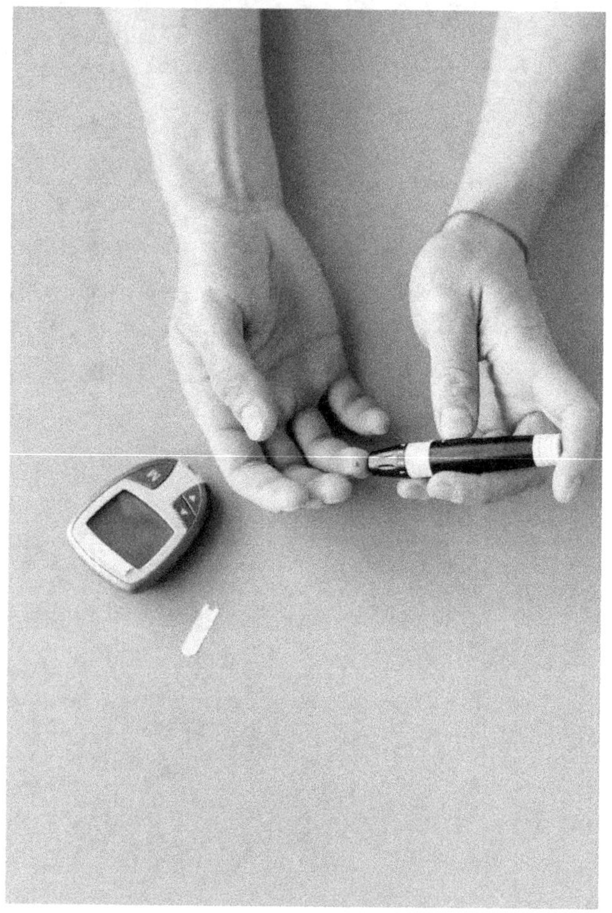

The following are some of the potential health hazards associated with high or low blood sugar levels:

Hyperglycemia (high blood sugar)

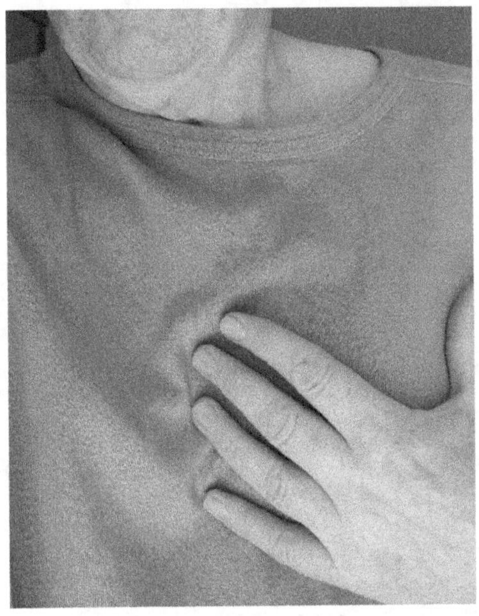

1. **Diabetes Complications:** Having high blood sugar levels for an extended period of time increases the risk of having diabetes complications such as heart disease, stroke, kidney disease, nerve damage (neuropathy), eye

damage (retinopathy), and circulation difficulties.

2. **Diabetic Ketoacidosis (DKA):** Excessively high blood sugar levels in persons with type 1 diabetes or poorly controlled type 2 diabetes can result in DKA. This is a dangerous condition that demands quick medical attention and can be fatal if left untreated.

3. **Hyperosmolar Hyperglycemic State (HHS):** This syndrome, which is more common in persons with type 2 diabetes, arises when blood sugar levels climb to dangerously high levels, causing severe dehydration, confusion, and even coma. HHS is a medical emergency as well.

Hypoglycemia (Low Blood Sugar)

1. **Seizures:** Severe hypoglycemia can produce seizures, which can be fatal and demand rapid medical intervention.

2. **Impaired Driving Skills:** Low blood sugar levels can alter reaction times, focus, and judgment, making driving or operating machinery unsafe.

3. **Accidental Risk:** Hypoglycemia can induce symptoms such as weakness, blurred vision, and poor coordination, which raises the risk of accidents, falls, and injuries.

4. **Cognitive Impairment:** When blood sugar levels fall too low, brain function is affected, resulting in confusion, trouble concentrating, dizziness, and, in severe cases, loss of consciousness

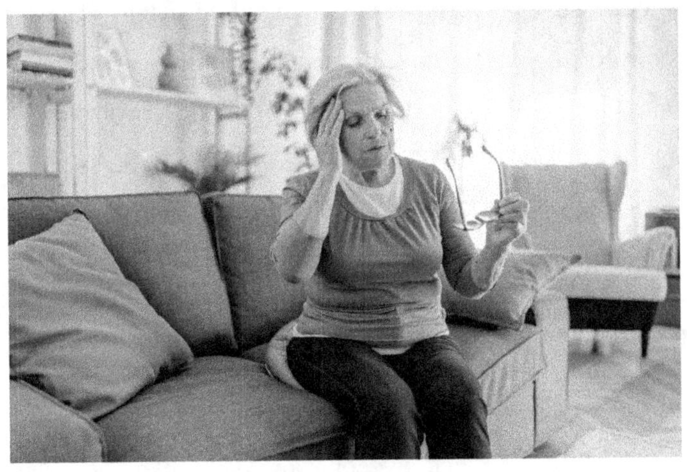

Chapter 2: The Impact of Blood Sugar Imbalance

The link between blood sugar imbalance and chronic health conditions

The link between blood sugar imbalance and chronic health challenges is well recognized, with chronic high blood sugar levels (hyperglycemia) being strongly connected to the development and progression of a number of illnesses. Diabetes is the most well-known chronic health risk connected with blood sugar imbalance, yet blood sugar dysregulation can also influence other conditions. Understanding this link is critical for prevention, management, and general health.

1. **Diabetes**: Diabetes is a chronic condition characterized by consistently high blood sugar

levels. Type 1 diabetes happens when the body does not create enough insulin, but type 2 diabetes is caused by insulin resistance, which occurs when the body does not efficiently use insulin. Diabetes unchecked can cause a range of issues, including cardiovascular disease, renal disease, nerve damage, eye problems, and an increased risk of infection.

2. **Cardiovascular Disease:** High blood sugar levels lead to the development of cardiovascular disease. Prolonged hyperglycemia destroys blood vessels, creating atherosclerosis (the formation of fatty deposits in the arteries), which raises the risk of heart attacks, strokes, and peripheral arterial disease.

3. **Obesity:** Obesity is characterized by blood sugar anomalies, specifically high blood sugar levels, which can contribute to weight gain and obesity. Elevated blood sugar increases fat storage, and obesity is a substantial risk factor for the development of many chronic diseases, including heart disease, type 2 diabetes, and some types of cancer.

4. **Metabolic syndrome:** This is a set of disorders that usually occur simultaneously, including high blood pressure, high blood sugar levels, abnormal cholesterol levels, and extra abdominal fat. A crucial component of metabolic syndrome is blood sugar imbalance, specifically insulin resistance. Metabolic syndrome increases the risk of cardiovascular disease, type 2 diabetes, and stroke.

5. **Chronic Kidney Disease:** High blood sugar levels that persist can injure the kidneys, resulting in chronic kidney disease. The kidneys filter waste from the blood, but high blood sugar levels could strain their function and limit their capacity to filter adequately.

6. **Nerve Damage:** Diabetic neuropathy is a condition caused by continuously increased blood sugar levels. Nerve injury most typically affects the peripheral nerves and can cause tingling, numbness, discomfort, and loss of sensation in the extremities. It can also have an influence on other organs and systems, such as the digestive and cardiovascular systems.

7. **Eye Problems:** Elevated blood sugar levels can damage the blood vessels in the eyes, leading to diabetic retinopathy, the main cause of blindness in people. It can also boost the risk of other eye problems like cataracts and glaucoma.

8. **Immune System Impairment:** High blood sugar levels can weaken the immune system, making it less effective in battling infections. This raises the risk of infections, poor wound healing, and susceptibility to numerous illnesses.

9. **Cognitive Decline:** High blood sugar levels that are unmanaged have been related to an increased risk of cognitive decline, dementia, and Alzheimer's disease. Blood sugar imbalances can impair brain function and contribute to memory issues and cognitive decline.

10. **Chronic Inflammation:** Elevated blood sugar levels contribute to the body's chronic inflammation. Chronic inflammation has been related to a range of chronic diseases, including heart disease, diabetes, autoimmune disorders, and various malignancies.

Exploring the link between blood sugar and weight gain

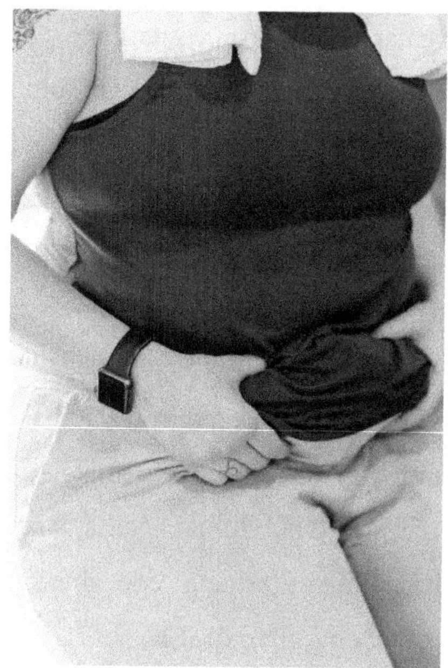

The link between blood sugar and weight rise is complex and multidimensional, but blood sugar levels can affect weight gain and contribute to the development of obesity in a variety of ways.

1. **Insulin and Fat Storage:** When blood sugar levels rise, the body creates insulin to help transport glucose into cells for energy generation or storage. Insulin is also involved in fat metabolism regulation. Continuously high blood

sugar levels and insulin surges, on the other hand, can increase the storage of extra glucose as fat. This can lead to weight gain and fat accumulation, particularly in the belly region.

2. **Increased Appetite and Cravings:** Blood sugar changes may have an impact on hunger and appetite regulation. Consuming high-sugar or high-carbohydrate foods can cause a quick increase in blood sugar levels, followed by a decrease. This decrease causes hunger signals to be delivered, raising desires for sweet or carbohydrate-rich foods. These calorie-dense meals could contribute to weight gain over time.

3. **Impaired Satiety Signaling:** Blood sugar abnormalities can impair the body's ability to identify fullness and pleasure after eating. Foods having a high sugar or glycemic index can trigger a quick jump and subsequent dip in blood sugar levels, leading to increased appetite and a predisposition to overeat. This might lead to an increase in calorie consumption and weight gain.

4. **Insulin Resistance:** Prolonged high blood sugar levels can evolve into insulin resistance, a

condition in which cells become less receptive to insulin's activities. As a result, the body creates extra insulin to compensate, which may contribute to weight gain. Insulin resistance promotes fat accumulation and can increase hunger, particularly in high-sugar, high-calorie diets.

5. **Metabolic Syndrome:** Blood sugar abnormalities, particularly insulin resistance, are usually associated with metabolic syndrome, a collection of illnesses defined by high blood pressure, raised blood sugar levels, abnormal cholesterol levels, and extra belly fat. Metabolic syndrome raises the probability of gaining weight, becoming obese, and acquiring chronic conditions such as type 2 diabetes and cardiovascular disease.

6. **Disrupted Energy Balance:** Blood sugar abnormalities can affect overall energy balance, which is the link between energy intake (calories taken) and energy expenditure (calories burned). High blood sugar levels on a regular basis can upset this balance by increasing fat storage and

limiting the body's capacity to adequately burn stored fat for energy. This might contribute to weight gain and make it difficult to decrease weight.

Effects of uncontrolled blood sugar on energy levels, mood, and cognitive function

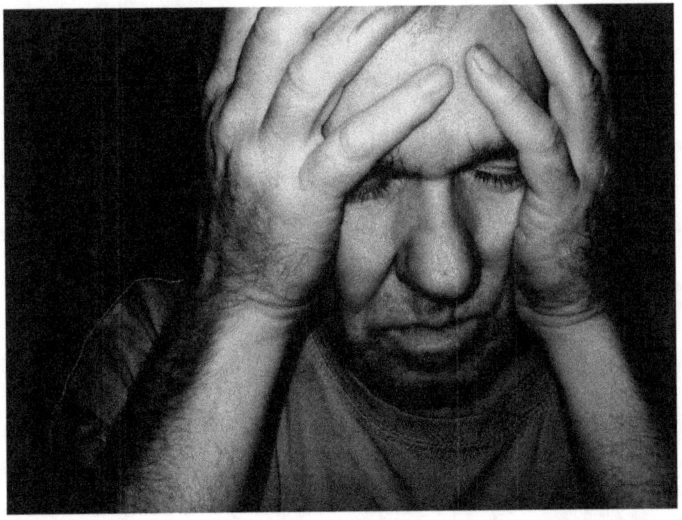

Uncontrolled blood sugar levels can have significant

implications for energy levels, emotions, and cognitive function, compromising both physical and mental health. Let's take a more in-depth look at these effects:

1. **Energy Levels:** Imagine waking up exhausted and bewildered after a long night. Unchecked, your blood sugar is out of control. You ride a rollercoaster of energy highs and lows throughout the day. High blood sugar levels can cause an initial spike of energy, followed by a decline as the body seeks to manage glucose. This energy dip leaves you exhausted, lethargic, and unable to function optimally. Maintaining productivity becomes a daily battle, and even routine jobs become challenging.

2. **Mood:** Imagine oneself angry, easily agitated, or experiencing quick mood fluctuations. These emotional changes can be induced by uncontrolled blood sugar levels. High blood sugar levels can interfere with the generation of serotonin, a neurotransmitter that aids in mood control. As your blood sugar rises and falls, so does your mood, creating feelings of anger,

stress, and even sorrow. Chronic emotional volatility can impair relationships and jeopardize general well-being.

3. **Cognitive Function:** Consider attempting to focus on a task or solve an issue but finding your mind foggy and scattered. Uncontrolled blood sugar levels have the potential to impair cognitive function and mental clarity. High blood sugar levels can limit blood circulation to the brain, lowering cognitive skills like focus, memory, and decision-making. It becomes difficult to remember information, maintain organization, and effectively process thoughts. This cognitive impairment can interfere with academic or professional performance and make even simple mental tasks appear challenging.

4. **Brain Fog:** Visualize yourself in a deep fog, where your ideas become murky and elusive. Uncontrolled blood sugar levels can contribute to "brain fog," a symptom. It looks like a mental fog has descended, affecting your capacity to think effectively, recollect information, and articulate thoughts. Concentration becomes

elusive, resulting in lower production and increased dissatisfaction.

5. **Mental Tiredness:** Imagine the weight of mental tiredness seeping in on you. Uncontrolled blood sugar levels can contribute to mental weariness, in which even easy mental tasks become psychologically tiring. Concentration becomes harder to sustain, and mental energy swiftly dissipates. This mental weariness relates to impaired cognitive function and decreases overall productivity and performance.

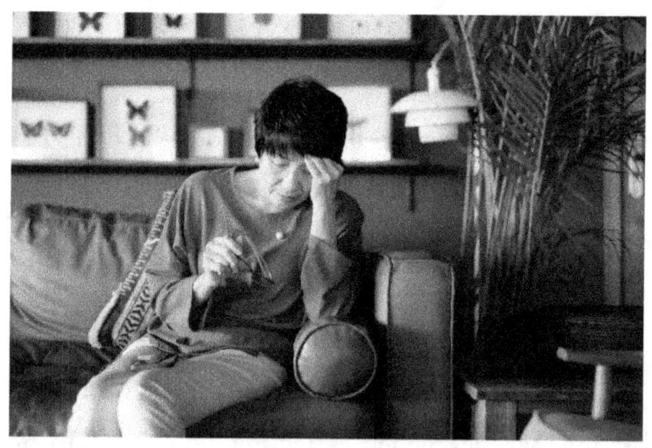

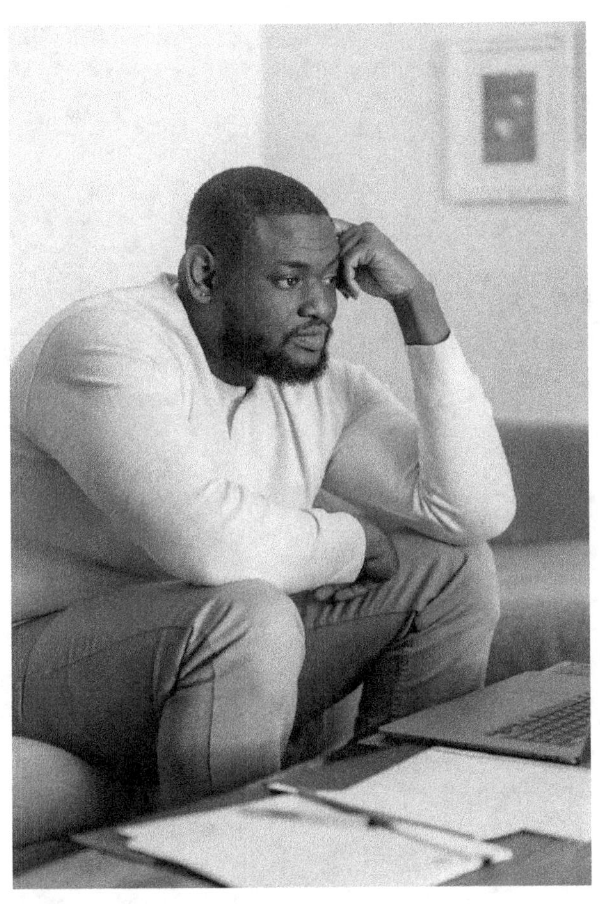

Chapter 3: Identifying Blood Sugar Imbalance

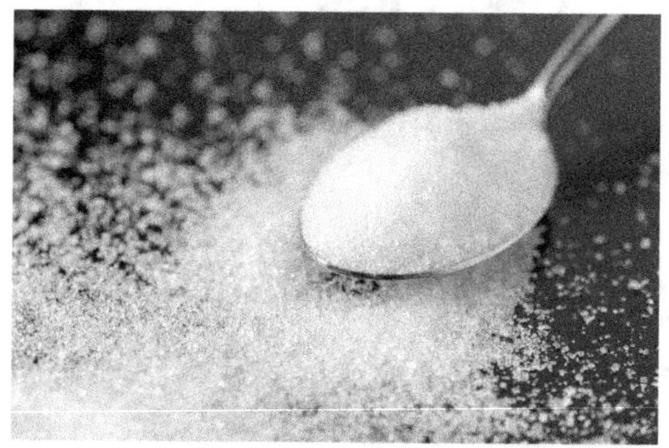

Blood sugar imbalance must be identified by monitoring and recognizing the signs and symptoms associated with high or low blood sugar levels.

Symptoms and signs of high blood sugar (hyperglycemia)

High blood sugar, also known as hyperglycemia, results when there is an excess of glucose circulating in the bloodstream. Here are some of the most typical indications and symptoms of high blood sugar:

1. **Increased thirst:** Excessive thirst, also known as polydipsia, is a symptom of high blood sugar. The body strives to compensate for the higher glucose levels by indicating the need for additional water.

2. **Frequent urination:** High blood sugar promotes increased urine flow, resulting in frequent urination (polyuria). The kidneys work harder to eliminate extra glucose from the bloodstream, resulting in a higher volume of urine.

3. **Weariness and weakness**: Hyperglycemia can produce weariness, exhaustion, and a lack of vitality. Because of insulin resistance or insufficient insulin synthesis, the body's cells may not be utilizing glucose for energy adequately.

4. **Blurred vision:** High blood sugar levels can cause changes in the shape of your eyes' lenses, resulting in blurred vision. This symptom

normally goes away once blood sugar levels are controlled.

5. **Increased Hunger:** You may have extended hunger (polyphagia) even having high blood sugar levels. It is likely that the cells are not acquiring enough glucose, resulting in increased hunger and food cravings.

6. **Rapid and unexplained weight loss:** Excessive blood sugar can induce rapid and unexplained weight loss. Due to insufficient glucose utilization, the body may begin to break down muscle tissue and store fat as an alternative energy source.

7. **Dry mouth and dry skin:** High blood sugar levels can cause dehydration, resulting in a dry mouth and dry, itchy skin. Increased urine flow leads the body to shed fluids.

8. **Infections:** High blood sugar levels damage the immune system, making you more prone to infections. In persons with uncontrolled hyperglycemia, recurrent urinary tract infections, yeast infections, and skin infections are prevalent.

9. **Slow wound healing:** Diabetes inhibits the body's capacity to heal wounds. Minor wounds, scratches, or sores may take longer to heal, and the risk of infection is enhanced in these places.

10. **Confusion:** Hyperglycemia can impair cognitive function, causing confusion, trouble concentrating, and poor decision-making. This symptom happens more commonly in severe situations of high blood sugar.

Symptoms and signs of low blood sugar (hypoglycemia)

Low blood sugar, generally known as hypoglycemia, occurs when blood glucose levels fall below normal. Here are some common low blood sugar symptoms and signs:

1. **Shakiness and trembling:** Feeling unstable or trembling is one of the earliest indicators of hypoglycemia. You may notice trembling in

your hands, legs, or voice as a result of the body's response to low glucose levels.

2. **Perspiration:** Hypoglycemia commonly induces perspiration, even if the surroundings are not heated. You may notice cold, clammy skin and profuse perspiration.

3. **Rapid heartbeat:** Low blood sugar can induce an increase in heart rate, resulting in palpitations or the sense that your heart is racing.

4. **Dizziness and lightheadedness:** Dizziness and lightheadedness are common signs of hypoglycemia. It can cause problems with your balance and coordination, making you feel uneasy.

5. **Hunger and nausea:** Low blood sugar levels can cause acute hunger and an overwhelming desire to eat. Some people may also feel queasy or have an upset stomach.

6. **Excessive weariness, weakness:** Excessive weariness, weakness, and an overall lack of vitality can arise from hypoglycemia. You can feel physically and psychologically weary.

7. **Concentration difficulties:** Low blood sugar levels can disrupt cognitive function, making it difficult to concentrate, focus, or think clearly. You may have mental disorientation or difficulties executing things.

8. **Irritability and mood swings:** Hypoglycemia can have an effect on your mood and emotions. You might feel angered, anxious, or nervous. Some people may experience mood swings or heightened emotional sensitivity.

9. **Headaches:** In some people, low blood sugar levels can produce headaches or migraines. The strength and duration of these headaches can vary.

10. **Blurred vision:** Temporary blurred vision or abnormalities in vision could develop following episodes of hypoglycemia. This symptom normally goes away as blood sugar levels return to normal.

Understanding the importance of regular blood sugar monitoring

Regular blood sugar monitoring is essential for controlling and maintaining optimal health, particularly for persons with diabetes or at risk of developing blood sugar irregularities. Here are some of the key reasons why frequent blood sugar monitoring is essential:

1. **Diabetes control:** For diabetic patients, regular blood sugar monitoring is crucial for efficient diabetes control. It gives crucial information about how well blood sugar levels are controlled, allowing for timely modifications in medication, diet, and lifestyle choices. Monitoring aids in the avoidance of problems and the maintenance of stable blood sugar levels within the target range indicated by healthcare specialists.

2. **Treatment Modifications:** Regular blood sugar monitoring delivers crucial information on the success of diabetic medications such as medicines, insulin therapy, and lifestyle adjustments. Individuals and healthcare providers can make educated judgments about prescription dosages, scheduling, and treatment regimens by tracking blood sugar levels.

3. **Identification of Hypoglycemia and Hyperglycemia:** Blood sugar monitoring aids in the identification of hypoglycemia (low blood sugar) and hyperglycemia (high blood sugar). Detecting these imbalances early enables swift corrective action to avoid complications. Prompt treatment can prevent severe hypoglycemia symptoms like loss of consciousness and minimize the chance of hyperglycemia crises like diabetic ketoacidosis.

4. **Lifestyle Management:** Regular blood sugar monitoring enables individuals to make informed lifestyle decisions. Individuals can better understand how these variables affect their blood sugar control by researching how their

blood sugar levels respond to altering diets, physical exercise, stress, and other events. This understanding enables people to make necessary modifications to their nutrition, exercise routine, stress management approaches, and overall lifestyle.

5. **Early diagnosis and intervention:** Regular blood sugar monitoring can detect potential blood sugar problems even before symptoms arise. This early detection enables proactive treatment to avoid the progression of prediabetes to diabetes or to successfully control diabetes. In high-risk individuals, early intervention through lifestyle changes can often postpone or prevent the onset of diabetes.

6. **Feedback and Motivation:** Blood sugar monitoring on a frequent basis provides quick feedback on the influence of lifestyle decisions and medication adherence on blood sugar levels. Seeing the direct association between behaviors and blood sugar levels can act as an incentive to make positive adjustments and stay dedicated to diabetes control.

7. **Collaborative Care:** Blood sugar monitoring findings are crucial for healthcare practitioners to examine therapy performance, make educated decisions, and provide personalized suggestions. Individuals and their healthcare teams benefit from regular monitoring because it develops efficient communication and shared decision-making.

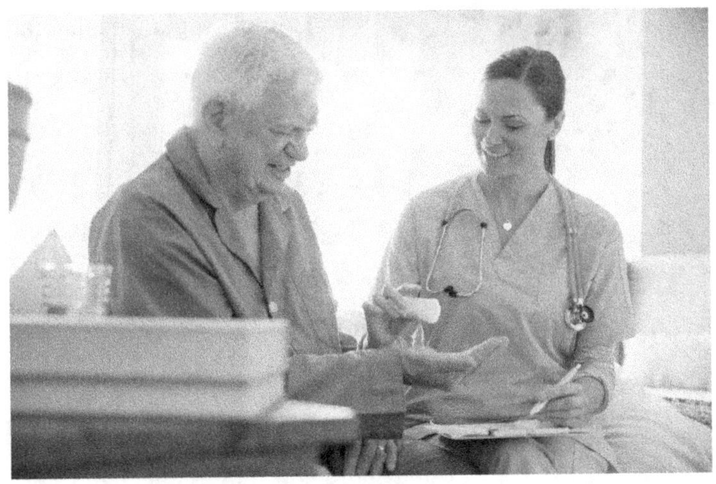

Chapter 4: Nutrition for Blood Sugar Balance

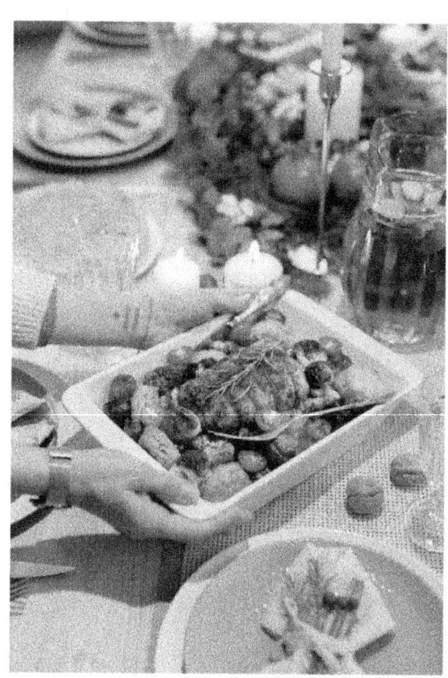

The meals we eat have a huge impact on achieving and maintaining blood sugar balance. Proper nutrition is vital for regulating blood sugar levels and supporting overall health. Here are some crucial factors of eating for blood sugar balance:

1. **Balanced Macronutrients:** A well-balanced diet comprises a spectrum of carbohydrates, proteins, and fats. The quality and quantity of these macronutrients, on the other hand, are critical for blood sugar regulation. Complex carbohydrates, such as whole grains, legumes,

and vegetables, are digested more slowly, resulting in a steady flow of glucose into the bloodstream. Combine carbohydrates with lean proteins and healthy fats to slow digestion and deliver long-lasting energy.

2. **Fiber-Rich Foods:** Consuming an adequate amount of dietary fiber is advantageous to blood sugar regulation. Fiber limits glucose absorption and contributes to more stable blood sugar levels. Choose fiber-rich foods such as fruits and vegetables, whole grains, nuts, and seeds.

3. **The glycemic index (GI):** This is a statistic that categorizes carbohydrates based on their influence on blood sugar levels. Low GI foods digest and absorb more slowly, resulting in a more gradual rise in blood sugar. Low GI diets such as non-starchy vegetables, legumes, and whole grains should be favored, whereas high GI meals such as sugary snacks, white bread, and refined grains should be avoided.

4. **Meal control:** Managing meal proportions is crucial for blood sugar regulation. Overeating, even with wholesome foods, can result in an

excessive intake of carbohydrates, leading to blood sugar rises. Consider portion sizes and try for balanced meals that incorporate a variety of nutrient-dense foods.

5. **Regular Meal Timing:** Meal timing is crucial for blood sugar management. Meal spacing throughout the day improves blood sugar regulation and prevents extreme changes. Avoid skipping meals because it could induce blood sugar decreases and subsequent overeating or bad food choices.

6. **Healthy Snacking:** Snacking between meals can assist maintain blood sugar homeostasis. Snack on items that blend carbohydrates, proteins, or healthy fats, such as an apple with nut butter or Greek yogurt with berries. These combinations give sustained energy by delaying the passage of glucose into the circulation.

7. **Hydration:** Staying well hydrated promotes both overall health and blood sugar regulation. Water controls metabolism, digestion, and nutrition delivery. Drink lots of water throughout

the day and avoid sugary beverages, which can trigger blood sugar rises.

8. **Mindful Eating:** This requires paying attention to hunger cues, eating carefully, and remaining present throughout meals. This technique develops a healthier relationship with food, fosters portion control, and prevents overeating.

9. **Individualized Approach:** It's crucial to realize that everyone's dietary needs are different. Age, activity level, underlying health conditions, and medications can all have an impact on blood sugar sensitivity to varied diets. A registered dietitian or healthcare professional can provide tailored counsel and support for optimizing nutrition and blood sugar control.

By implementing these concepts into your eating habits, you may be able to maintain your blood sugar balance, enhance general health, and lower your risk of diseases related to blood sugar irregularities. Remember that achieving long-term nutritional adjustments is a lengthy process, so concentrate on consistency and long-term excellent eating habits.

The role of carbohydrates, proteins, and fats in blood sugar regulation

Carbohydrates, proteins, and fats each have a unique role in blood sugar regulation. Understanding their impact is vital for maintaining stable blood sugar levels. Here's a thorough overview of their roles:

1. Carbohydrates

Carbohydrates are the principal source of glucose, the main form of sugar needed by the body for energy. When ingested, carbohydrates are broken down into glucose and taken into the bloodstream. The type and quantity of carbohydrates taken can drastically impact blood sugar levels.

- **Simple Carbohydrates**

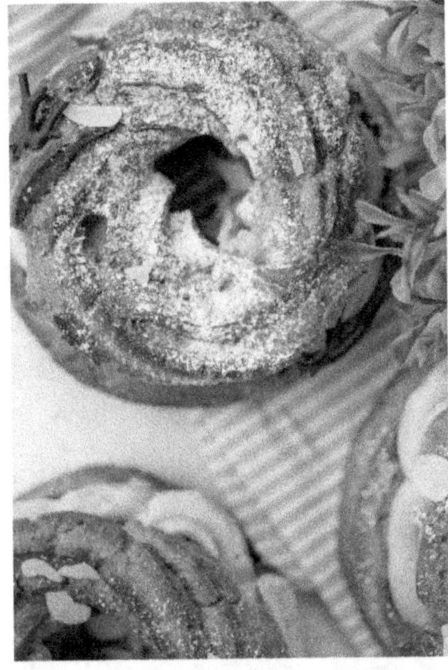

These are easily absorbed and induce a sudden surge in blood sugar levels. Foods such as refined sugars, sugary beverages, candy, and white bread fall into this group. It's crucial to take simple carbohydrates in moderation.

- **Complex carbohydrates**

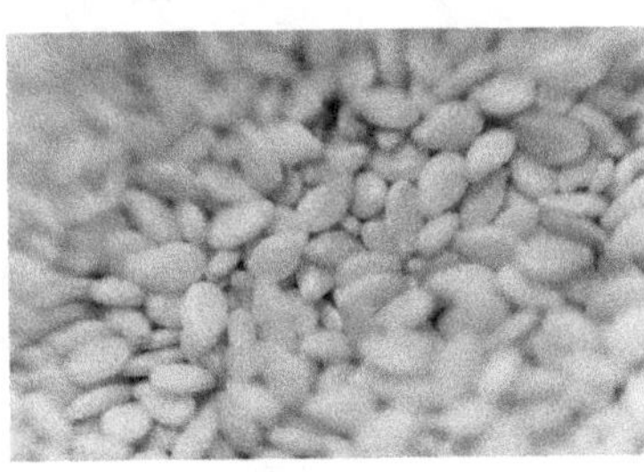

Complex carbohydrates consist of fiber, starches, and whole grains. They are digested more slowly, resulting in a gradual and constant release of glucose into the bloodstream. Examples are whole grains, legumes, fruits, and vegetables. These carbohydrates give a longer sustained source of energy and have a reduced impact on blood sugar levels.

2. Proteins

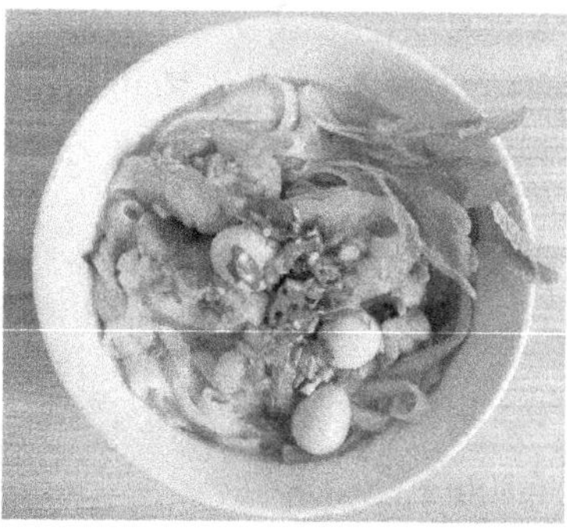

Proteins have a function in blood sugar management by providing a more prolonged release of glucose compared to carbohydrates. When eaten, proteins are broken down into amino acids, which can be turned into glucose through a process called gluconeogenesis. This procedure helps maintain blood sugar levels during periods of fasting or minimal carbohydrate intake.

Including protein in meals and snacks can help slow down the digestion and absorption of carbohydrates, minimizing rapid spikes in blood sugar levels. Good sources of protein include lean meats, poultry, fish, eggs, dairy products, legumes, and plant-based proteins such as tofu and tempeh.

3. Fats

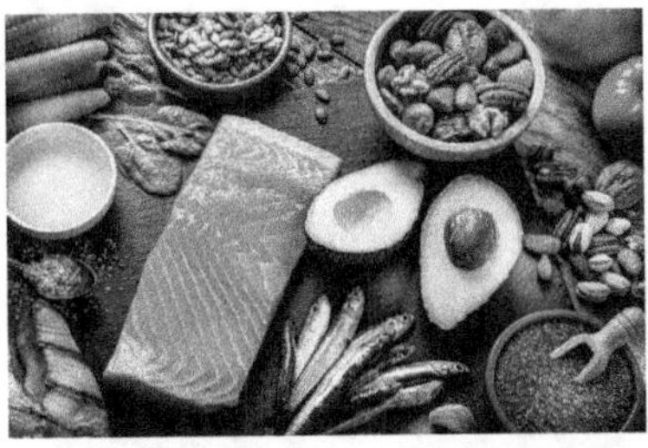

Dietary fats have a low direct impact on blood sugar levels since they do not include carbohydrates and have little effect on insulin secretion. However, lipids play a critical function in satiety and slowing down the digestion and absorption of carbohydrates.

Including healthy fats in meals can help manage blood sugar by delivering a sense of fullness and reducing the overall glycemic load of a meal. Examples of healthful fats include avocados, nuts, seeds, olive oil, fatty fish, and nut butter. It's vital to choose sources of unsaturated fats while limiting saturated and trans fats, as they can have detrimental health impacts.

Balancing Macronutrients

To maintain blood sugar balance, it's vital to aim for a balanced combination of carbohydrates, proteins, and fats in each meal. This can be achieved by:

- Prioritizing complex carbohydrates from whole grains, fruits, and vegetables.
- Including lean proteins from sources including poultry, fish, lentils, and plant-based proteins.
- Incorporating healthy fats from sources such as avocados, almonds, and olive oil.

The percentage of each macronutrient may vary depending on individual demands, health conditions, and activity levels. Working with a qualified dietitian or healthcare professional can assist identify tailored macronutrient ratios for optimal blood sugar regulation.

It's worth mentioning that the timing and amount sizes of meals can influence blood sugar management. Consistency in meal time and portion control are key for maintaining stable blood sugar levels throughout the day.

A balanced diet that contains proper portions of carbohydrates, proteins, and fats can lead to better blood sugar regulation, energy levels, and general health.

Glycemic index and glycemic load: understanding their impact on blood sugar

Understanding the concepts of glycemic index (GI) and glycemic load (GL) can provide significant insights into how different foods affect blood sugar levels. Let's look at these theories and their consequences for blood sugar regulation:

1. **Glycemic Index (GI)**

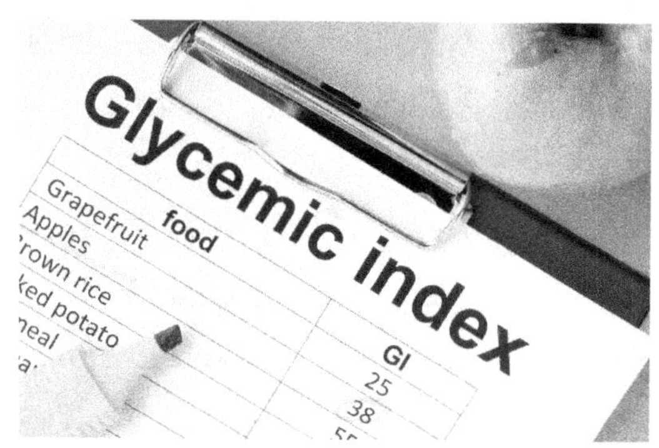

The glycemic index is a scale that compares carbohydrate-containing meals to pure glucose or white bread (both of which have a GI of 100). Foods with a high GI digest rapidly and generate a sudden increase in blood sugar levels, whereas foods with a low GI absorb slowly and create a persistent rise in blood sugar.

The following is a general breakdown of GI ranges:

- GI of 55 or less
- GI Medium: 56-69
- High GI: 70 or above

Most non-starchy vegetables, legumes, whole grains, and some fruits have a low GI. These foods promote a slower and more persistent release of glucose into the bloodstream, resulting in more stable blood sugar levels.

Some fruits, whole wheat products, and basmati rice have a medium GI. White bread, white rice, sugary drinks, and processed snacks are examples of high GI foods. Excessive eating of high GI meals can produce fast spikes in blood sugar levels, potentially leading to insulin resistance and an increased risk of chronic diseases.

2. **Glycemic Load (GL)**

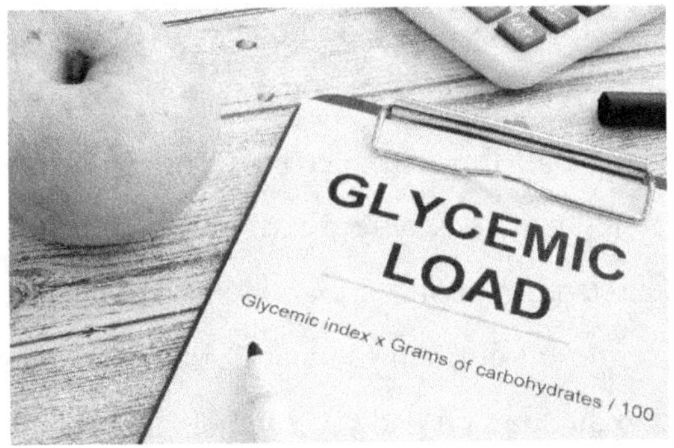

While GI delivers significant information about how foods affect blood sugar levels, it does not address portion quantities. Glycemic load considers both the quality (GI) and quantity of carbohydrates. It studies the overall influence of a certain amount of food on blood sugar levels.

The GL of a food is calculated by multiplying the grams of accessible carbohydrates in it by its GI and then dividing by 100. The following is a breakdown of GL ranges:

- Low GL: 10 or fewer
- 11-19 Medium GL
- High GL: 20 or above

Low GL foods have a modest effect on blood sugar levels, whereas high GL foods can cause large increases. Watermelon, for example, has a high GI but a low GL since it contains very few carbohydrates per serving. Understanding both GI and GL assists consumers to make more informed food choices. Choosing meals with low to medium GI and GL can help maintain more stable blood sugar levels throughout the day, increasing general health and minimizing the risk of insulin resistance, diabetes, and other chronic illnesses.

It is crucial to note, however, that the GI and GL should not be the primary determining criteria in meal planning. Other aspects to consider are general nutrition, meal proportions, and individual health goals.

A certified dietitian or healthcare expert can provide specific advice on integrating low-GI and low-GL items into a balanced diet for optimal blood sugar regulation and overall well-being.

Identifying and avoiding hidden sugars in processed foods

Identifying and avoiding hidden sugars in processed meals is crucial for maintaining stable blood sugar levels and overall health. Many processed foods have added sugars, which may contribute to blood sugar abnormalities if consumed in excess. Here are some strategies to help you find and avoid hidden sugars:

1. **Read food labels:** Begin by reading the ingredient list on food labels. Look for common names for added sugars including sucrose, high fructose corn syrup, dextrose, maltose, and syrup. Keep in mind that ingredients are offered in descending order by weight, so if a type of sugar is listed at or near the top, it suggests a higher sugar concentration.

2. **Look for alternative names:** Sugar can emerge under different names, hence it is vital to be aware of these aliases. Cane juice, agave nectar, honey, molasses, fruit juice concentrate, and evaporated cane juice are all names that refer to added sugars.

3. **Look for sugar-related phrases:** Some processed goods may contain statements like "no added sugar," "sugar-free," or "low sugar" on their package. However, it is still necessary to check the nutrition information panel and ingredient list for any hidden sugars. These terms may signify that different sweeteners or sugar substitutes were utilized.

4. **Be wary of "healthy" foods:** Even ostensibly nutritious processed items, such as granola bars, flavored yogurt, or breakfast cereals, can contain large amounts of added sugars. To determine the sugar content, always look at the nutrition data.

5. **Examine the carbohydrate content:** The overall carbohydrate value on the nutrition label includes both naturally occurring sugars and added sugars. To find hidden sugars, compare the total carbohydrate content to the quantity of dietary fiber. If the carbohydrate percentage is much higher than the fiber content, it suggests a higher sugar level.

6. **Choose whole foods:** Eating entire, unprocessed foods including fruits, vegetables, lean meats, and whole grains is an effective method to limit hidden sugar intake. These meals are often lower in added sugars and contain critical minerals and fiber.

7. **Cook and prepare meals at home:** By cooking from scratch, you have more control over the ingredients and can limit the quantity of added sugars in your diet. When necessary, use natural

sweeteners such as fruits, spices (cinnamon, vanilla), or small amounts of honey or maple syrup.

8. **Be mindful of condiments and sauces:** Pay attention to the sugar content of condiments, dressings, sauces, and marinades. These typically contain hidden sugars. Consider crafting your own versions with healthier components or selecting ones with no added sweeteners.

9. **Limit sugary beverages:** Sugary beverages such as soda, fruit juices, energy drinks, and flavored coffees or teas can be high in hidden sugars. Instead, pick water, unsweetened tea, or infused water.

10. **Be a responsible consumer:** Maintain vigilance and make well-informed decisions. Don't get sucked in by misleading marketing claims. Before purchasing or eating processed items, study the nutrition data and ingredient list.

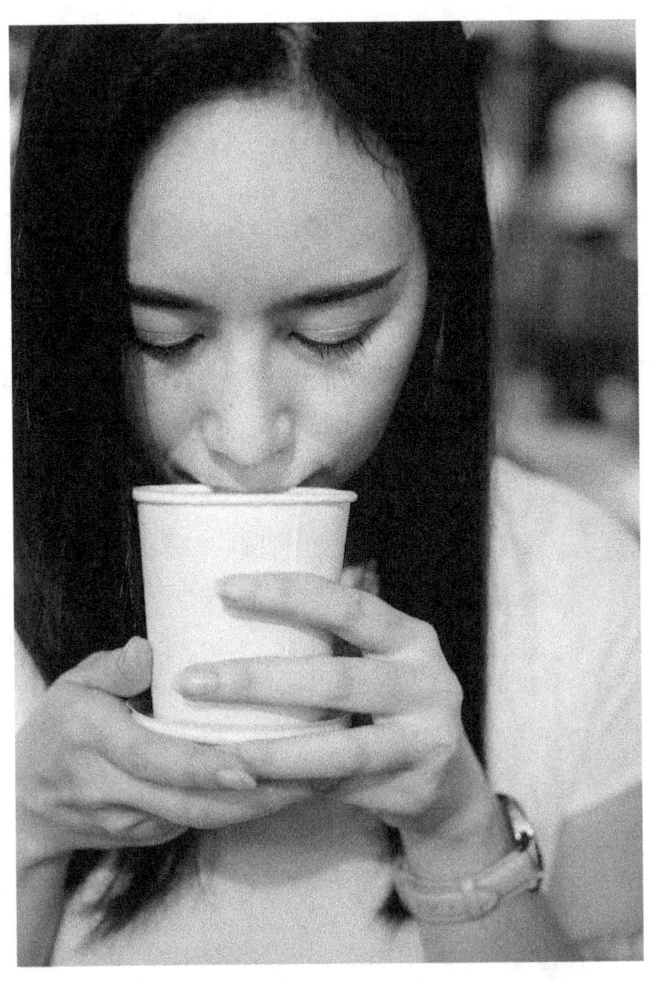

Chapter 5: Lifestyle Strategies for Blood Sugar Management

Implementing lifestyle strategies is essential for efficiently regulating blood sugar levels. These tactics concentrate on numerous areas of daily life, such as diet, physical activity, stress management, and sleep. Individuals can enhance their blood sugar control and overall health by embracing these lifestyle modifications. Let's have a look at some vivid lifestyle tips for blood sugar control:

1. **Balanced and Healthy Eating**

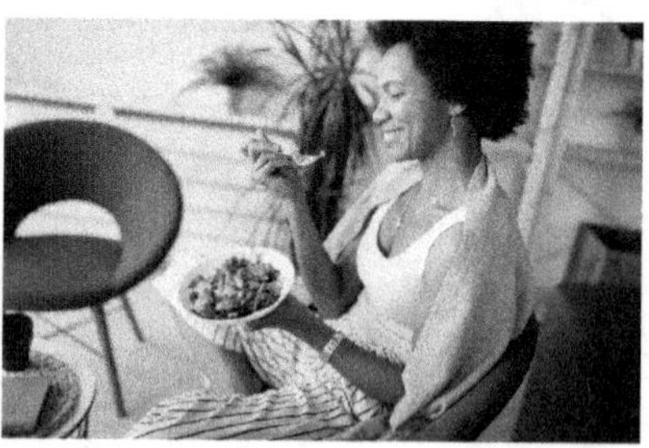

Adopting a balanced and healthy food plan is vital for blood sugar regulation. Emphasize complete, unprocessed foods such as fruits and vegetables, whole grains, lean meats, and healthy fats. To avoid blood sugar spikes, limit meal quantities and distribute carbohydrates evenly throughout the day. In addition, to help manage blood sugar levels, emphasize foods with a low glycemic index and glycemic load.

2. **Regular Physical Activity**

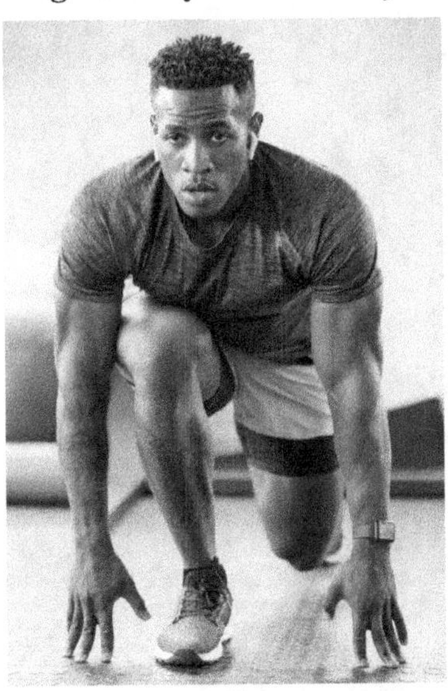

Regular physical activity offers numerous advantages for blood sugar management. Exercise decreases blood sugar levels, boosts insulin sensitivity, and improves metabolic health overall. Choose activities that you enjoy, such as brisk walking, cycling, dancing, or swimming, and aim for at least 150 minutes a week of moderate-intensity activity. Consult your healthcare practitioner to identify the greatest effective fitness regimen for your unique circumstances.

3. **Stress Reduction**

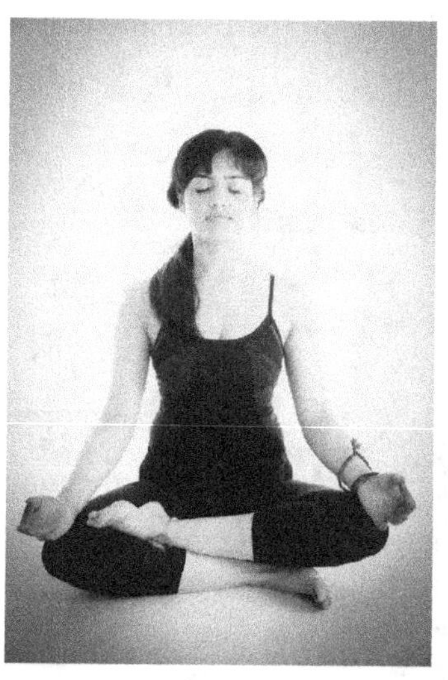

Chronic stress may contribute to blood sugar abnormalities. Incorporating stress management practices can be effective. Explore soothing activities such as yoga, meditation, deep breathing exercises, mindfulness techniques, or hobbies. Prioritize self-care and develop healthy techniques to handle stress to help keep blood sugar levels steady.

4. **Quality sleep**

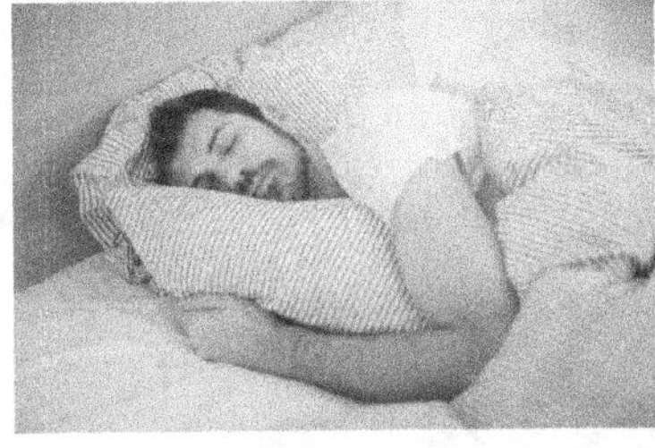

Adequate and restorative sleep is necessary for blood sugar regulation. Sleep deprivation can disturb the hormonal balance, lower insulin sensitivity, and contribute to cravings and overeating. Opt for 7-9 hours of sleep every night. To increase sleep quality, stick to a consistent sleep schedule, maintain a pleasant resting environment, and practice suitable sleep hygiene behaviors.

5. **Hydration**

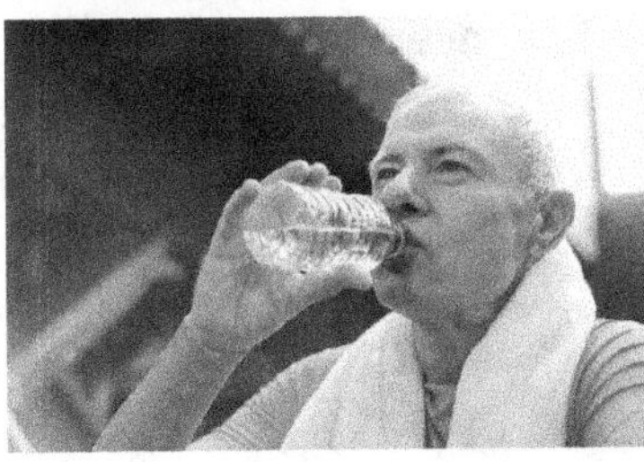

Adequate hydration is crucial for blood sugar regulation. Water promotes optimal biological functioning, such as metabolism and digestion. Aim to drink enough water throughout the day and limit your intake of sugary beverages. Carry a water bottle to remind yourself to stay hydrated.

6. **Regular monitoring of blood sugar levels**

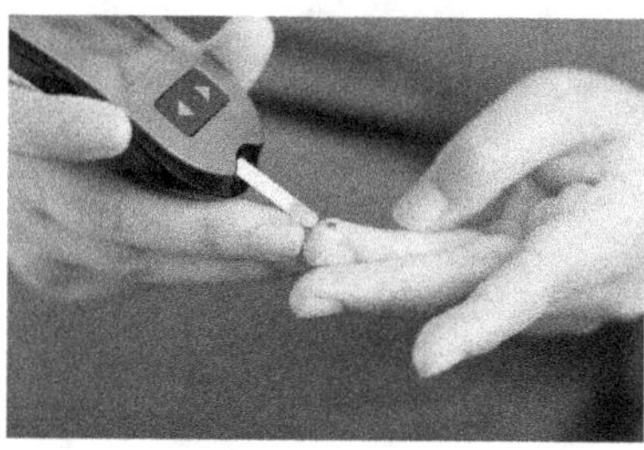

This is crucial for optimal control. Follow your healthcare provider's advice for how frequently and when to monitor your blood sugar. Monitoring allows you to discover how your body reacts to various foods, activities, and medications, allowing you to make better-informed lifestyle decisions.

7. **Medication Management**

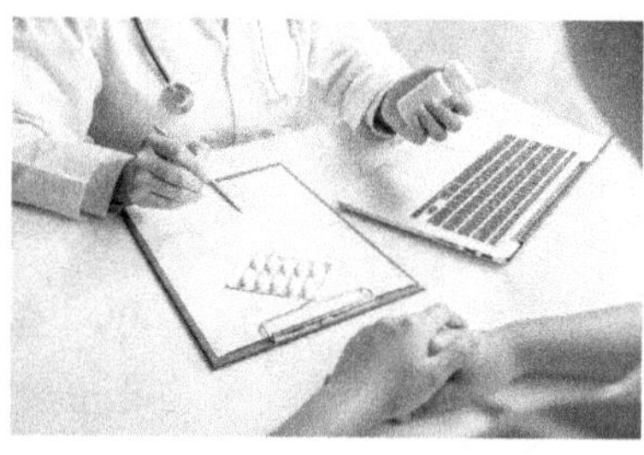

If you are prescribed medication for blood sugar control, it is vital that you take it exactly as advised by your healthcare physician. Follow the dosage and time recommendations, and report any concerns or unpleasant effects to your healthcare professional. Proper medication distribution, coupled with lifestyle adjustments, can assist optimize blood sugar control.

8. **Support Network**

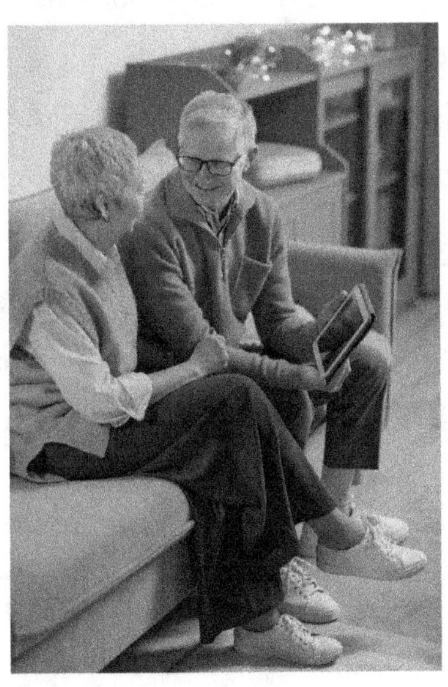

Building a support network might be highly effective in lowering blood sugar levels. Seek help from family, friends, or support groups who understand your predicament. Share your concerns, achievements, and anxieties with them, and consider joining diabetic education programs or online groups for extra knowledge and support.

The value of regular physical activity in blood sugar regulation

Regular physical activity is vital for blood sugar management and overall health in persons who have or are at risk of developing blood sugar disorders. Here are some in-depth observations regarding the requirement of frequent physical activity for blood sugar control:

1. **Increased Insulin Sensitivity:** Physical exercise enhances insulin sensitivity, allowing your body to use insulin more effectively. When you work out, your muscles demand glucose for energy. This boosts glucose absorption into cells without relying exclusively on insulin. As a result, engaging in regular physical activity can help lower blood sugar levels and minimize the risk of insulin resistance.

2. **Improved Glucose homeostasis:** Physical activity improves blood sugar homeostasis by

boosting the uptake and use of glucose by your muscles. It aids in the depletion of glycogen stores in the muscles, which stimulates your body to replenish these stores with glucose from the bloodstream. This approach aids in the maintenance of steady blood sugar levels.

3. **Weight Control:** Physical activity enhances weight control, which is crucial for blood sugar regulation. Regular exercise aids in the burning of calories, the development of lean muscle mass, and the improvement of body composition. Maintaining a healthy weight lowers the chance of having type 2 diabetes and aids in the management of blood sugar levels.

4. **Increased Energy Expenditure:** Physical exercise increases energy expenditure, which results in better calorie utilization. When you exercise at a moderate to high intensity, your body uses glucose as fuel. This can aid blood sugar stability by reducing blood sugar levels during and after exercise.

5. **Cardiovascular Health:** Regular physical exercise improves the cardiovascular system,

minimizing the risk of heart disease, which is commonly related to blood sugar abnormalities. Exercise boosts circulation, decreases blood pressure, lowers bad cholesterol (LDL), and raises good cholesterol (HDL), all of which lead to better overall cardiovascular health.

6. **Stress Reduction:** Physical activity is an excellent stress reducer. Stress can create blood sugar abnormalities by stimulating hormonal reactions that boost blood sugar levels. Regular exercise can assist to reduce stress, enhance relaxation, and improve general mental health.

7. **Long-Term Blood Sugar Control:** Consistent physical exercise is associated with long-term blood sugar control. Regular exercise can help persons at risk avoid or postpone the onset of type 2 diabetes. Physical activity is an important component of diabetes therapy for adults with diabetes and can lead to better blood sugar management.

8. **Overall Health Benefits:** Regular physical activity provides various other health advantages. It supports healthy body weight,

enhances cardiovascular fitness, increases bone density, strengthens muscles, improves immune function, promotes better sleep, and improves overall quality of life.

Aim for a combination of aerobic and strength training exercises (such as weightlifting or resistance training) to maximize the benefits of physical activity for blood sugar control. Before beginning a new exercise plan, check with your healthcare professional, especially if you have any current medical concerns.

Effective stress management tactics for blood sugar normalization

Individuals with blood sugar issues or diabetes benefit substantially from stress management approaches. Stress increases the release of chemicals such as cortisol and adrenaline, which can increase blood sugar levels. Effective stress management can assist to prevent blood sugar spikes and support improved overall blood sugar management. Consider the following helpful stress management methods:

1. **Regular Physical Activity**: This is a good stress reducer. Walking, jogging, cycling, dancing, or yoga may help alleviate tension. Exercise increases the release of endorphins, which are natural mood boosters, and improves relaxation.

2. **Deep Breathing and Relaxation Techniques:** Deep breathing techniques, such as diaphragmatic breathing or progressive muscular relaxation, can assist activate the body's relaxation response and reduce stress. Take calm, deep breaths, focusing on your abdomen's rise and fall. To enhance relaxation and stress reduction, you can also attempt guided imagery, meditation, or mindfulness activities.

3. **Prioritization and Time Management:** Effective time management can help minimize stress. Set acceptable goals and divide them into small parts. By carefully managing your

schedule, you can avoid feeling overwhelmed and reduce stress.

4. **Healthy Lifestyle Practices:** Adopting appropriate living practices can help with stress management greatly. Make sure you're getting enough sleep, eating a balanced diet, and avoiding stimulants like caffeine and alcohol. These practices boost general health and help your body cope with stress.

5. **Social Support:** Seek assistance from family, friends, or support groups. Talking about your difficulties with people or conducting activities with loved ones can provide emotional support and help relieve tension. Sharing one's feelings and experiences can be comforting and assist to develop a sense of community.

6. **Relaxation Techniques:** Discover soothing strategies that work for you. Listening to calm music, taking a warm bath, practicing aromatherapy, or engaging in hobbies that offer you joy and help you unwind are all examples of ways to relax.

7. **Cognitive-behavioral approaches:** Approaches such as cognitive restructuring and positive self-talk, can benefit stress management by modifying negative thought patterns and creating a more positive view. Replace negative thinking with realistic and hopeful affirmations.

8. **Make time for self-care a priority**: Reading, hobbies, spending time in nature, or self-reflection are all activities that can provide you delight and help you relax. Stress management necessitates that you take care of your emotional and mental well-being.

9. **Getting Professional Help:** If stress becomes unbearable or persists despite your efforts, you may consider receiving professional assistance. A therapist or counselor can guide you in building effective stress management methods that are personalized to your needs.

Sleep's Significance and Impact on blood sugar regulation

Sleep is necessary for optimal blood sugar management and general metabolic health. Adequate and restorative sleep is vital for persons who have blood sugar difficulties or diabetes.

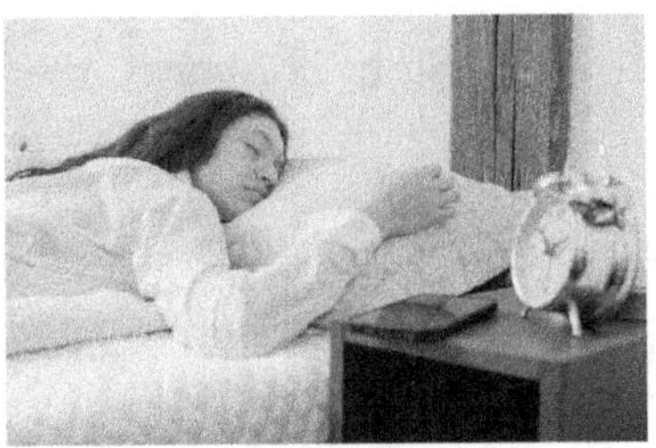

Here's a complete look at sleep and its impact on blood sugar regulation:

1. **Insulin Sensitivity:** Sleep deprivation or poor sleep quality may affect insulin sensitivity. When you don't get enough sleep, your body's capacity to effectively utilize insulin declines.

Over time, this can result in greater blood sugar levels and insulin resistance.

2. **Glucose Metabolism:** The body conducts many metabolic activities when sleeping, including glucose metabolism. Sleep enables your body to replenish and regulate blood glucose levels. Adequate sleep promotes glucose metabolism, decreasing blood sugar swings.

3. **Hormonal Regulation:** Sleep is directly linked to the regulation of hormones involved in blood sugar management. Sleep deprivation can disturb hormone balances such as cortisol, ghrelin, and leptin, all of which have involvement in appetite regulation, glucose metabolism, and insulin sensitivity. Disruptions in these hormones can lead to increased hunger, cravings for high-sugar foods, and blood sugar regulation difficulties.

4. **Circadian Rhythm:** Sleep is an integral component of the body's circadian cycle, which influences different physiological activities such as blood sugar management. Circadian cycle irregularities, such as irregular sleep patterns or

sleep interruptions, can result in blood sugar imbalances and an increased risk of insulin resistance.

5. **Overnight Fasting phase:** While sleeping, you enter an overnight fasting phase during which you normally go without eating for several hours. This extended fasting phase benefits blood sugar regulation by enabling insulin levels to drop and ensuring the liver maintains a consistent flow of glucose into the bloodstream. Sufficient sleep duration promotes constant blood sugar levels and supports the overnight fasting phase.

6. **Appetite and Cravings:** Sleep deprivation can have an influence on appetite-regulating hormones, resulting in increased hunger and cravings for high-calorie, sugary meals. This can lead to overeating and blood sugar disorders. Adequate sleep aids in the regulation of appetite hormones, reducing the probability of overeating and making bad food choices.

7. **Weight Management:** Lack of sleep has been linked to weight gain and obesity, both of which

are risk factors for blood sugar abnormalities. Poor sleep can disturb the balance of hunger-regulating hormones, increase appetite, and contribute to overeating. Inadequate sleep can also contribute to weariness and decreased motivation for physical activity, changing weight management, and blood sugar control.

8. **Overall Well-Being:** Adequate sleep is vital for physical and mental health. Sleep deprivation can contribute to stress, emotional disorders, and difficulties with everyday duties. Stress and poor mental health may have an indirect effect on blood sugar management and make it more difficult to keep beneficial lifestyle choices.

Breaking sedentary habits and sustaining an active lifestyle

It is vital to break sedentary habits and maintain an active lifestyle for overall health and blood sugar control. Here are some techniques for incorporating more activity and overcoming sedentary habits:

1. **Set Realistic Goals:** Begin by defining feasible goals that correlate to your current fitness level and lifestyle. Attempt to gradually raise your level of activity over time. Begin with simple, achievable goals, such as taking short daily walks or introducing shorter exercise sessions into your regimen.

2. **Find things you enjoy doing:** Do activities you enjoy doing. Choose activities that match your hobbies, such as dancing, swimming, cycling, hiking, or sports. When you enjoy a workout, you are more likely to persevere with it and incorporate it into your daily routine.

3. **Make It a Habit:** Breaking sedentary behaviors demands consistency. Make physical activity an inevitable part of your everyday routine. Make time for exercise and approach it as a vital appointment with yourself. Begin with a low frequency, such as three times per week, and gradually increase as your momentum grows.

4. **Incorporate Movement Into Your Regular Routine:** Look for techniques to incorporate movement into your regular activities. Take the stairs instead of the elevator, walk or pedal small distances, stand up and stretch during breaks, and arrange walking meetings rather than sitting in a conference room. These modest modifications might add up and help prevent inactivity.

5. **Use Activity Trackers or Applications:** Consider using activity trackers or mobile applications that track your daily steps, distance, or exercise time. These tools can motivate you, track your progress, and remind you to remain active throughout the day.

6. **Set Regular Breaks:** Take regular movement breaks to break up long periods of sitting. Set an alarm for every hour to get up and stretch, go for a short stroll, or perform some simple exercises. Even a few minutes of movement can have a major impact on your overall activity level.

7. **Find a Partner for Accountability:** Join forces with a friend, family member, or coworker who

shares your desire to live an active lifestyle. Working out with or being accountable to someone can enhance motivation and make physical activity more enjoyable.

8. **Try New Things:** Trying new things keeps things interesting and reduces boredom. Experiment with numerous activities and exercise modalities to find out what you enjoy the most. Consider taking group fitness courses, joining a sports league, or discovering new outdoor activities.

9. **Make it Social:** Include physical activity in social settings. Instead of meeting for coffee, go for a walk or hike together. Organize physical activities with friends or family, such as bike trips, beach volleyball, or dance lessons. In this manner, you can maintain social contacts while remaining active.

10. **Be Aware of Sedentary Habits:** Pay attention to sedentary habits and look for ways to improve them. Limit excessive screen time, such as watching television or using cell phones, and replace it with more active exercises. Stand or

walk when conversing on the phone, do short workouts during TV commercials, and if possible, utilize a standing desk.

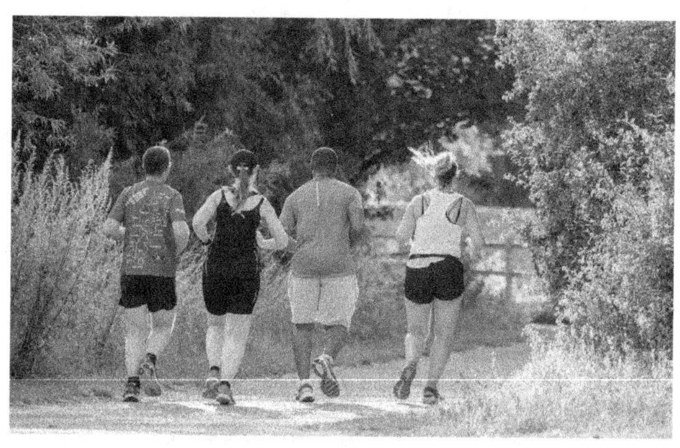

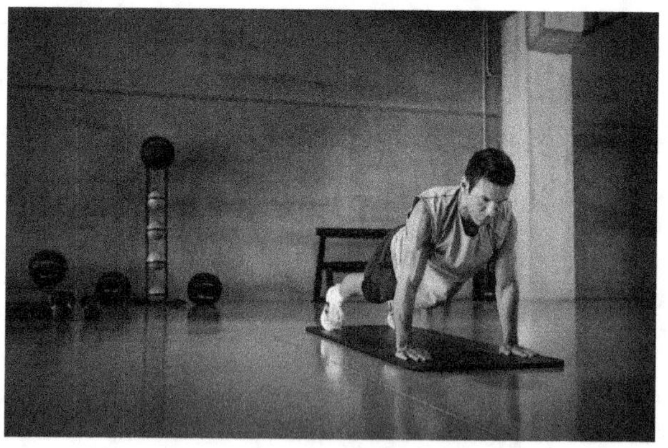

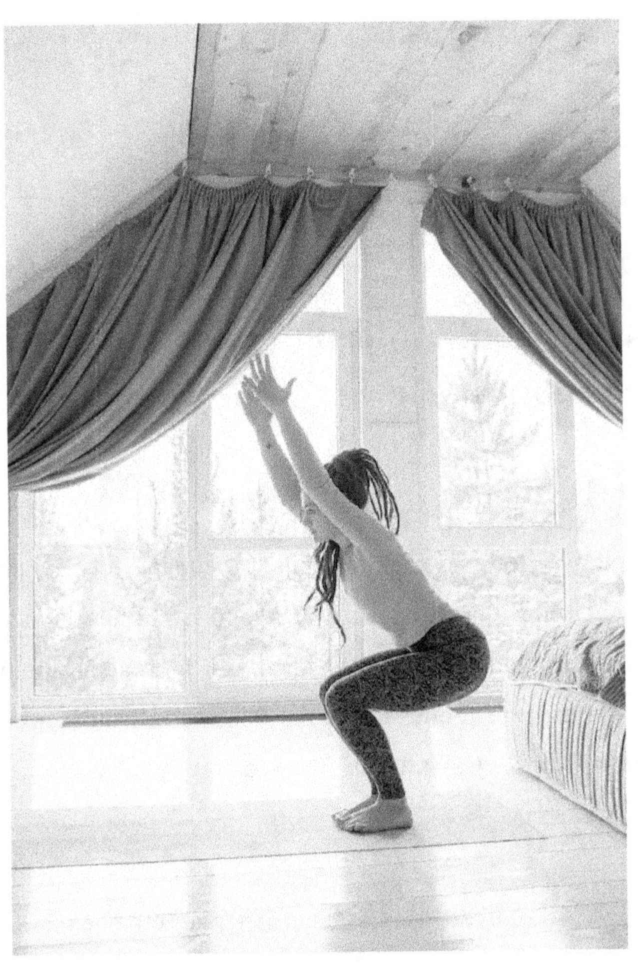

Chapter 6: The Glucose Revolution Code Diet Plan

A full explanation of the Glucose Revolution Code Diet plan

The Glucose Revolution Code diet plan is a complete strategy for regulating blood sugar levels and maintaining general health. It supports eating balanced meals, reducing carbohydrates, and consuming nutrient-dense foods. The following is a full summary of the Glucose Revolution Code eating plan's essential components:

1. **Balanced Meals:** The diet plan emphasizes the requirement of eating balanced meals that contain a range of lean proteins, healthy fats, and complex carbohydrates. This equilibrium reduces glucose digestion and absorption,

resulting in less rapid spikes in blood sugar levels. Chicken, turkey, salmon, tofu, and lentils are all examples of lean proteins. Avocados, almonds, seeds, and olive oil are all fantastic sources of healthy fats.

2. **Carbohydrate Control:** Managing carbohydrate consumption is a vital component of the Glucose Revolution Code diet plan. It advocates eating carbohydrates with a low glycemic index (GI), which implies they have a slower effect on blood sugar levels. Low GI diets include non-starchy vegetables, whole grains, legumes, and the majority of fruits. This strategy contributes to more constant blood sugar levels throughout the day.

3. **Portion management:** Portion control is emphasized in order to avoid overeating and maintain a balanced nutrient intake. The diet plan specifies the ideal protein, carbohydrate, and fat consumption proportions. Measuring and measuring food may initially assist people in becoming acquainted with acceptable portion proportions.

4. **Glycemic Load Awareness:** The Glucose Revolution Code diet plan includes the notion of glycemic load (GL) in addition to the glycemic index. GL considers both the quality and quantity of carbohydrates in a dish. It supports consumers in making better-informed selections by considering both the glycemic index and the amount of carbohydrates consumed.

5. **Nutrient-Dense Foods:** The diet plan promotes the consumption of nutrient-dense foods, which supply necessary vitamins, minerals, and antioxidants. This includes a variety of colorful fruits and vegetables that are high in fiber and phytonutrients. Fish, poultry, tofu, and lentils are also advised as lean proteins. In moderation, healthy fats like avocados, almonds, seeds, and olive oil are used.

6. **Hydration:** Staying hydrated is vital for overall health and blood sugar regulation. The Glucose Revolution Code diet plan stresses drinking water throughout the day and avoiding sugary beverages. Drinking water can help you stay

hydrated and assist your body's natural processes.

7. **Mealtime:** Eating regularly is recommended to keep blood sugar levels stable. Eating at regular times throughout the day helps to avoid long periods of fasting and acute hunger, which can lead to poor food choices and blood sugar abnormalities.

8. **Mindful Eating:** The Glucose Revolution Code diet plan supports mindful eating, which includes paying attention to hunger and fullness indicators, eating carefully, and savoring each meal. Mindful eating supports people in building a healthy relationship with food, reducing overeating, and fostering better digestion.

9. **Physical Activity:** Alongside dietary considerations, the diet plan emphasizes the importance of regular physical activity. Engaging in aerobic exercises, strength training, or other activities that increase heart rate and promote muscle strength can help improve insulin sensitivity, enhance blood sugar control, and support overall health.

10. **Individualization:** The Glucose Revolution Code diet plan realizes that everyone's needs are different. It encourages customization based on tastes, health concerns, and lifestyle variables. A professional dietitian or healthcare specialist can provide specialized guidance and help.

Sample blood sugar-balancing meal plans and dishes

Here are a few sample meal plans and recipes designed to stabilize blood sugar levels:

Meal Plan 1

Breakfast

- Veggie omelet with egg whites, spinach, bell peppers, and tomatoes
- Whole grain toast with avocado spread
- Fresh berries

Snack:

- Greek yogurt with chopped almonds and a sprinkle of cinnamon

Lunch

- Grilled chicken breast with quinoa and steamed
- Mixed greens salad with cherry tomatoes, cucumber, and balsamic vinaigrette

Snack:

- Sliced bell peppers with hummus

Dinner

- Salmon baked with roasted asparagus and brown rice
- Side salad with mixed greens, sliced strawberries, feta cheese, and a light vinaigrette dressing

Snack:

- Apple slices with almond butter

Meal Plan 2

Breakfast

- Overnight oats made with rolled oats, almond milk, chia seeds, and topped with berries and a drizzle of honey
- Hard-boiled egg

Snack:

- Carrot sticks with almond butter

Lunch

Quinoa and black bean salad with mixed vegetables (e.g., diced bell peppers, corn, and cherry tomatoes) and a lime-cilantro dressing

Snack:

Greek yogurt garnished with chopped almonds and cinnamon

Dinner

- Grilled chicken breast with roasted Brussels sprouts and sweet potato wedges
- Steamed broccoli on the side

Snack:

- Celery sticks with guacamole

Recipes

1. Veggie Omelet

Ingredients

- Egg whites
- Spinach leaves
- Bell peppers (sliced)
- Tomatoes (diced)
- Salt and pepper to taste
- Cooking spray

Instructions

1. Coat a nonstick skillet with cooking spray and heat over medium heat.

2. Add the bell peppers and tomatoes to the skillet and sauté for a few minutes until slightly softened.

3. Cook until the spinach leaves are wilted.

4. In a separate bowl, whisk the egg whites with salt and pepper.

5. Pour the egg whites over the cooked vegetables in the skillet.

6. Prepare the omelet until the eggs are set, then fold it in half.

7. Transfer to a plate and serve.

2. Quinoa and Black Bean Salad

Ingredients

- Cooked quinoa
- Canned black beans (rinsed and drained)
- Mixed vegetables (e.g., diced bell peppers, corn, cherry tomatoes)
- Fresh cilantro (chopped)

- Lime juice
- Olive oil
- Salt and pepper to taste

Instructions

1. In a large bowl, combine the cooked quinoa, black beans, mixed vegetables, and cilantro.
2. In a separate small bowl, whisk together lime juice, olive oil, salt, and pepper to make the dressing.
3. To incorporate the dressing, pour it over the quinoa mixture and toss thoroughly.
4. Adjust seasoning if needed.
5. Serve chilled or at room temperature.

Remember to customize the portion sizes based on your individual needs and consult with a healthcare professional or registered dietitian for personalized guidance.

Including entire meals and nutrient-dense foods in your diet

A healthy eating plan demands you to incorporate full meals and nutrient-dense components into your diet. Whole foods are minimally processed and retain their natural state, delivering a variety of critical elements such as vitamins, minerals, fiber, and antioxidants. Here are various advantages and techniques to add whole foods and nutrient-dense foods into your diet:

1. **Nutrient Variety:** Whole foods contain a wide range of nutrients that are required for healthy health. You can guarantee that your body gets a wide range of vitamins, minerals, and other essential substances by integrating a variety of fruits, vegetables, whole grains, lean proteins, and healthy fats into your meals.

2. **Fiber-Rich Foods:** Whole foods like fruits, vegetables, whole grains, legumes, and nuts are high in fiber. Fiber improves digestion, controls blood sugar levels, and promotes heart health.

Incorporate a selection of fiber-rich foods into your meals and snacks.

3. **Reduced Sugars and Artificial Ingredients:** Whole foods are inherently low in added sugars, artificial additives, and preservatives. You can limit your exposure to potentially harmful elements while enhancing your general health by eating substantial meals.

4. **Improved Satiety and Weight Management:** Whole foods are usually more full and fulfilling than processed foods due to their higher fiber and nutrient content. You may help manage your appetite, maintain your weight, and lower your risks of overeating by including more whole foods in your diet.

5. **Cooking from Scratch:** Making meals at home with complete ingredients provides you more control over the quality of your food. It allows you to avoid hidden sugars, bad fats, and excess sodium that are typically found in processed foods. Experiment with easy recipes and culinary approaches to produce delectable and nutritious meals.

6. **Mindful Eating:** Including full foods enhances mindful eating. Paying attention to the scents, sensations, and delight that whole foods give can improve your entire dining experience and promote healthier food choices.

7. **Farmer's Markets & Local Produce:** To obtain fresh, locally grown produce, visit your local farmer's market or community-supported agriculture (CSA) program. These solutions frequently expand the range of complete meals available while also supporting local farmers and sustainable agriculture practices.

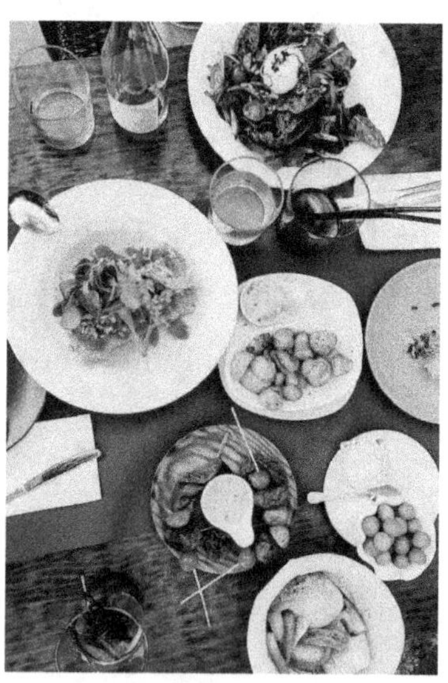

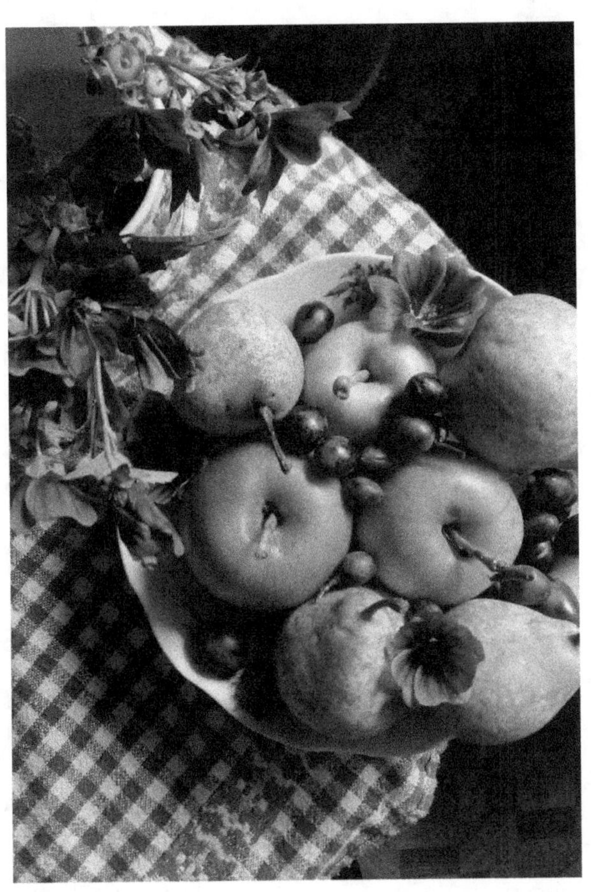

Chapter 7: Medications and Blood Sugar Management

Medications play a significant role in blood sugar management, especially for those who have diabetes or other conditions that cause blood sugar levels to vary. They are given to assist regulate blood sugar and prevent problems. The following is a list of common blood sugar management medications:

1. **Insulin:** Insulin is a hormone that regulates blood sugar levels by allowing cells to absorb glucose for energy. Individuals with type 1 and type 2 diabetes must utilize insulin injections or insulin pumps to control their blood sugar levels. There are several varieties of insulin, including rapid-acting, short-acting, intermediate-acting, and long-acting insulin, each with a different length and effect on blood sugar.

2. **Oral Diabetes medications:** Oral diabetes drugs are routinely used to help persons with type 2

diabetes maintain blood sugar levels. These drugs function in a variety of techniques, including increasing insulin production, enhancing insulin sensitivity, and lowering glucose synthesis in the liver. Metformin, sulfonylureas, thiazolidinediones, DPP-4 inhibitors, SGLT-2 inhibitors, and GLP-1 receptor agonists are examples of common oral diabetes treatments. Individual needs, medical history, and responsiveness to treatment will all impact which medication(s) are administered.

3. **Other Injectable medications:** In addition to insulin, injectable drugs are available for blood sugar management. GLP-1 receptor agonists, for example, are injectable drugs that enhance insulin secretion, decrease glucagon production, slow stomach emptying, and generate a feeling of fullness. They are frequently administered to persons with type 2 diabetes.

4. **Blood Sugar Regulators:** Some drugs, such as alpha-glucosidase inhibitors, assist regulate blood sugar levels by reducing carbohydrate breakdown and absorption in the intestines.

These drugs are regularly prescribed for persons with type 2 diabetes and can be taken orally.

5. **Medications for Underlying Illnesses:** When blood sugar imbalances are caused by underlying illnesses such as hormone imbalances or certain medications, treatment may include addressing the underlying cause. This may entail changing or stopping blood sugar-lowering drugs, as well as addressing the underlying issue.

To ensure that your medications and blood sugar management techniques are working effectively, it is vital to stick to the specified drug regimen, report any concerns or issues to your healthcare practitioner, and attend regular check-ups.

An Overview of typical blood sugar management drugs

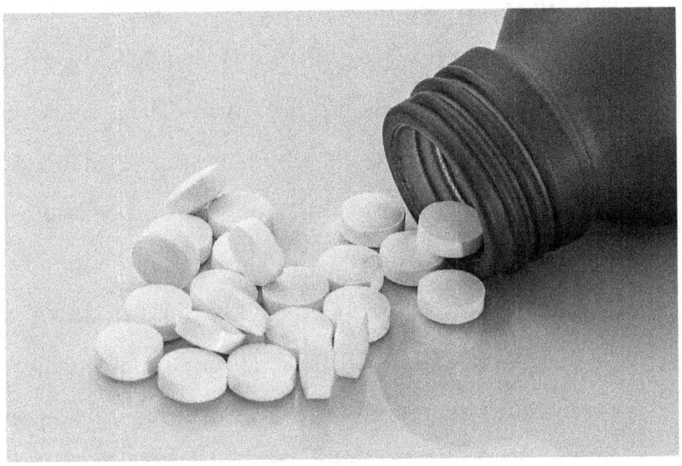

Common blood sugar control drugs include:

1. **Metformin:** Metformin is widely used as the first-line treatment for type 2 diabetes. It works by lowering glucose synthesis in the liver and boosting insulin sensitivity in the cells of the body. It could aid with weight loss.

2. **Sulfonylureas:** This class of drugs encourages the pancreas to generate more insulin. Glipizide,

glyburide, and glimepiride are a few examples. They are routinely administered to persons with type 2 diabetes.

3. **Thiazolidinediones (TZDs):** TZDs boost insulin sensitivity in cells while lowering glucose synthesis in the liver. They may be prescribed to persons who have type 2 diabetes. Pioglitazone and rosiglitazone are two examples.

4. **DPP-4 Inhibitors:** DPP-4 inhibitors operate by suppressing the enzyme that breaks down a hormone called GLP-1. These drugs enhance insulin secretion while lowering glucagon production by boosting GLP-1 levels. Sitagliptin, saxagliptin, and linagliptin are a few examples.

5. **SGLT-2 Inhibitors:** SGLT-2 inhibitors assist lower blood sugar levels by preventing glucose reabsorption in the kidneys, resulting in greater glucose excretion via urine. Canagliflozin, dapagliflozin, and empagliflozin are some examples.

6. **GLP-1 Receptor Agonists:** GLP-1 receptor agonists enhance insulin release, inhibit

glucagon synthesis, slow stomach emptying, and produce sensations of fullness. They may be prescribed to persons who have type 2 diabetes. Exenatide, liraglutide, and dulaglutide are a few examples.

7. **Insulin:** Insulin is a hormone that contributes to the regulation of blood sugar levels. It is used to treat persons with type 1 diabetes and those with type 2 diabetes who are unable to meet their blood sugar goals with oral drugs alone. Insulin comes in a variety of types, including rapid-acting, short-acting, intermediate-acting, and long-acting insulin, which can be supplied in various combinations based on individual needs.

Understanding the advantages and disadvantages of blood sugar management drugs

Medication is vital in the treatment of blood sugar levels in patients with diabetes or other illnesses that affect blood sugar levels. Here are some advantages and cons of utilizing blood sugar medication:

Advantages

1. **Blood Sugar Control:** Medications are created specifically to regulate blood sugar levels and assist keep them within a certain range. They can successfully regulate high blood sugar levels and avoid complications connected with high blood sugar.

2. **Diabetes management:** Medication is usually an important aspect of a diabetic's overall disease management plan. It aids in the management of symptoms, minimizes the risk of complications, and enhances quality of life.

3. **Access and Convenience:** Medications are widely available and simple to obtain. They can be taken orally, breathed, or delivered through injection, making them ideal for daily use.

4. **Complementary to Lifestyle Changes:** Medications operate in concert with lifestyle changes such as healthy food, frequent physical activity, and stress management to maintain optimal blood sugar control. They can provide further aid when lifestyle changes alone are insufficient.

5. **Preventive Effects:** Some blood sugar management drugs, such as metformin, have been discovered to have potential preventive effects on other diabetes-related health issues, such as cardiovascular disease.

Disadvantages

1. **Adverse effects:** Blood sugar control medicines, like any other drug, could have substantial negative effects. These can differ based on the medication and the individual's response. Gestural difficulties, weight gain, hypoglycemia (low blood sugar), and allergic responses are all

typical adverse effects. However, not everyone may develop adverse effects, and they are easily controlled with proper monitoring and correction.

2. **Individual Variability:** Because diverse people react differently to drugs, determining the exact prescription and dosage that is suited for an individual's specific needs may take trial and error. It may take some time to identify the most effective prescription or combination of drugs for optimal blood sugar control.

3. **Cost:** The cost of blood sugar management drugs varies depending on the type of prescription, insurance coverage, and healthcare system. Some prescriptions, particularly those for newer or brand-name medications, may be more expensive. It is vital to examine the financial ramifications and look at solutions for affordability, such as generic alternatives or patient support programs.

4. **Dependence:** Some people may become dependent on blood sugar-lowering drugs. While drugs are important, it is critical to realize the

importance of lifestyle adjustments and general self-care habits in efficiently maintaining blood sugar levels.

5. **Interaction with Other Pharmaceuticals:** Blood sugar control therapies may interact with other medications a person is taking, resulting in potential drug interactions. To ensure safe and effective management, it is vital to notify healthcare professionals about all prescriptions, including over-the-counter drugs and supplements.

The necessity of drug adherence and regular check-ups with healthcare experts

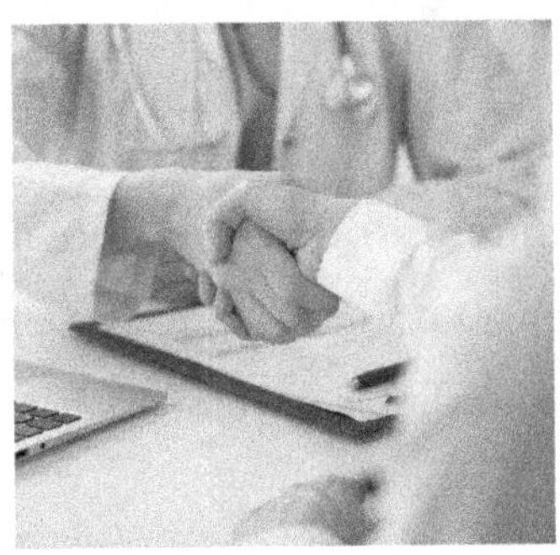

Adherence to medication and regular check-ups with healthcare professionals are necessary for good blood sugar management.

Here's a quick rundown of their significance:

1. **Medication Adherence:** It is vital to take medications as advised in order to maintain stable blood sugar levels. Adherence to the recommended treatment plan guarantees that the medications are operating as well as possible to manage blood sugar and limit the risk of complications. Skipping doses or failing to comply with the dosing guidelines can result in variable blood sugar levels, reducing therapeutic effectiveness.

2. **Consistent Blood Sugar Control:** Adherence to medication schedules aids in the maintenance of regular blood sugar management. Medications are meant to act during specified time periods, and taking them at the appropriate times preserves a regular amount of medication in the body, resulting in better management of blood sugar levels throughout the day.

3. **Complication Prevention:** Regular medication adherence can help avoid or postpone the onset of complications linked with high blood sugar

levels, such as heart disease, kidney disease, nerve damage, and eye issues. Medication that regularly manages blood sugar can considerably lower the incidence of these problems.

4. **Monitoring and Adjustment:** Regular check-ups with healthcare specialists, such as doctors or endocrinologists, allow you to assess the effectiveness of your medication and make any essential adjustments. To maintain optimal blood sugar management, healthcare experts can monitor blood sugar levels, assess medication adherence, and recommend any changes to the treatment regimen.

5. **Education and Support:** Healthcare professionals play a vital role in teaching and supporting patients regarding pharmaceutical consumption, potential side effects, and lifestyle changes. Regular check-ups allow people to ask questions, obtain advice on how to keep their blood sugar levels steady and learn about new improvements in diabetes care.

6. **Early detection of problems:** Regular check-ups allow healthcare experts to discover

any potential problems early on. They can keep an eye out for pharmaceutical side effects, examine the impact of medications on other health conditions, and notice any changes in blood sugar management requirements. Prompt intervention can help address difficulties and avoid problems.

7. **Customized Treatment Plans:** Regular check-ups enable healthcare practitioners to construct and alter customized treatment plans depending on the individual's changing needs and goals. They can improve outcomes and promote general well-being by altering prescription regimens, lifestyle suggestions, and blood sugar monitoring measures.

8. **Holistic Health Assessment:** Beyond blood sugar management, regular check-ups allow healthcare experts to analyze general health, including elements such as blood pressure, cholesterol levels, weight, and mental well-being. This thorough method covers any potential health issues and guarantees a holistic approach to total wellness.

Alternative approaches to medication, including natural remedies and supplements

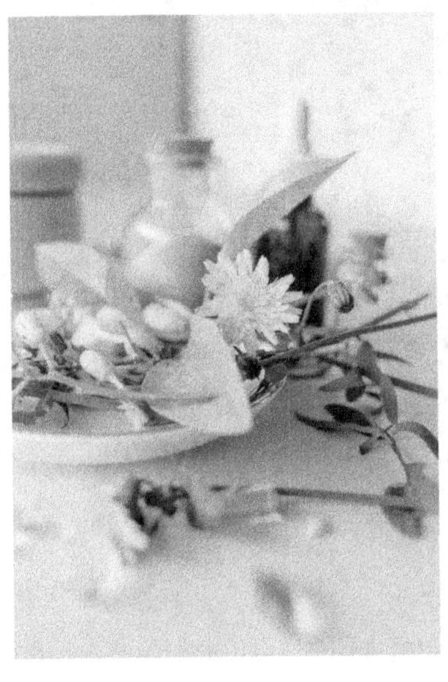

Alternative options to medication, including natural remedies and supplements, are often explored by folks looking for additional support in managing blood sugar levels. While these therapies may offer potential benefits, it's vital to approach them with caution and speak with a healthcare specialist. Here is a vivid review of alternate ways to medication for blood sugar management:

1. Herbal Remedies

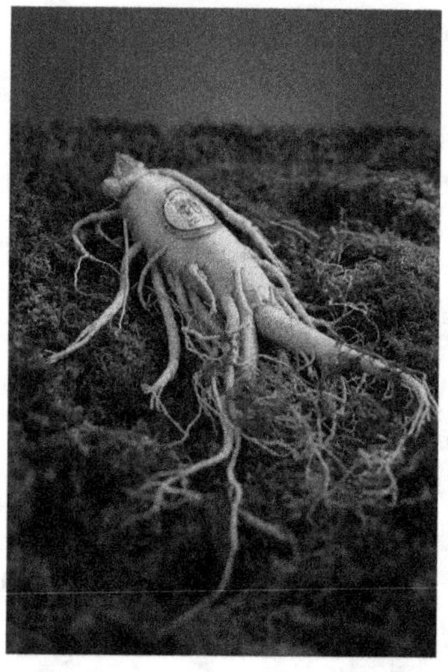

Certain herbs and botanicals have been traditionally used to support blood sugar control. Examples include cinnamon, fenugreek, ginseng, and bitter melon. These herbs may have qualities that may promote insulin sensitivity or regulate blood sugar levels. However, their efficiency could vary, and it's crucial to use them on the advice of a healthcare practitioner, as they can interfere with drugs or have harmful effects on certain folks.

2. Dietary Supplements

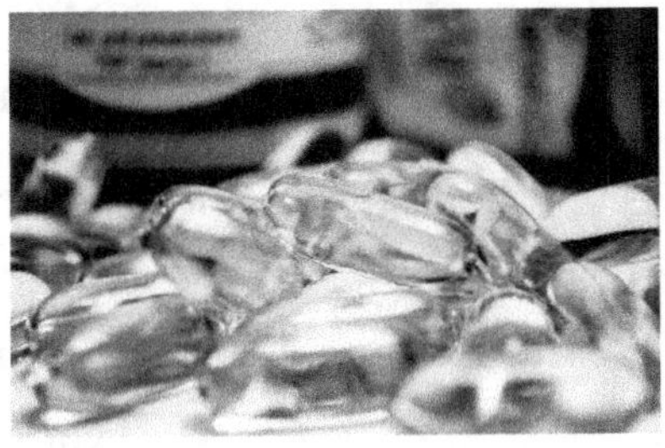 Some dietary supplements are available for blood sugar management. Examples include alpha-lipoic acid, chromium, magnesium, and omega-3 fatty acids. These drugs may have potential benefits in increasing insulin sensitivity or decreasing inflammation. However, their usefulness is still under investigation, and it's crucial to connect with a healthcare practitioner before integrating them into your routine. They should not replace prescribed drugs but rather be used as extra support.

3. **Mind-Body practices**

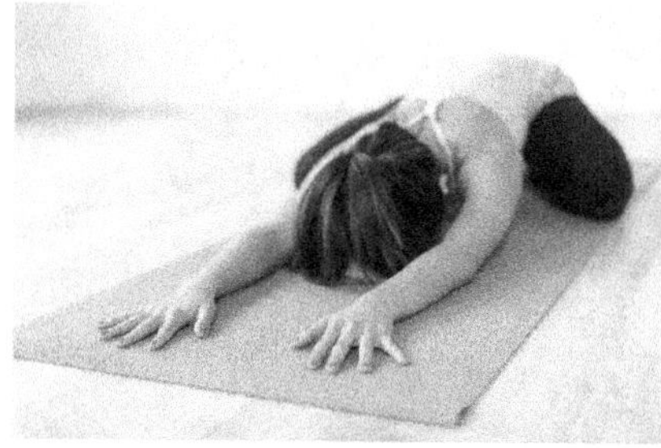

Stress management practices, such as meditation, yoga, and deep breathing exercises, can help regulate blood sugar levels indirectly. Chronic stress can compromise blood sugar control, hence these measures may help general well-being and assist in stable blood sugar management. However, they should not replace prescribed medications, and it's vital to talk with a healthcare practitioner to integrate these tactics into a comprehensive treatment plan.

4. Lifestyle modifications

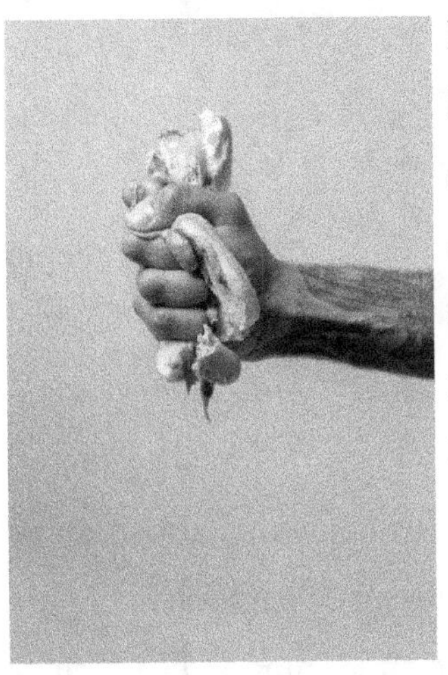

Making healthy lifestyle alterations can have a considerable impact on blood sugar management. Regular physical exercise, a balanced diet rich in whole foods, weight control, and sufficient sleep all have a role in stabilizing blood sugar levels. These lifestyle adjustments can complement medical therapy and may even reduce the need for medication in some cases. It's vital to contact a healthcare practitioner to design an individualized plan that integrates these lifestyle alterations efficiently.

5. Alternative Therapies

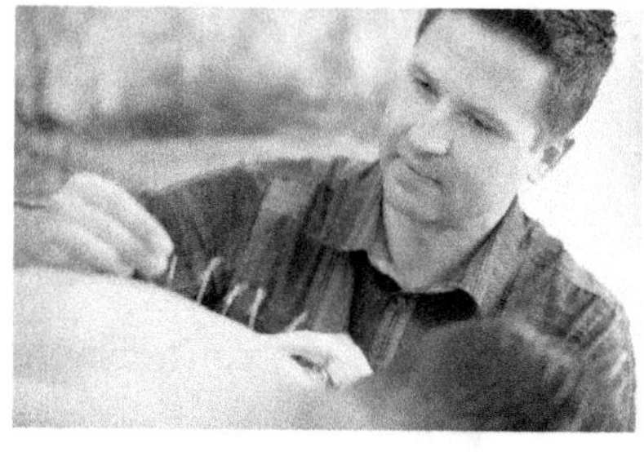

Some folks study alternative therapies like acupuncture, acupressure, or chiropractic care to support blood sugar management. These therapies may have a calming or pain-relieving effect, which might indirectly influence blood sugar levels. However, data supporting their unique influence on blood sugar control is minimal, and they should be provided with conventional medical care.

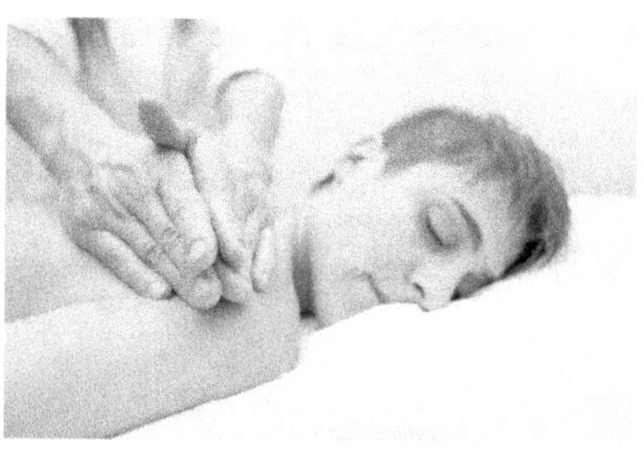

It's important to highlight that alternate techniques to treatment should never substitute approved drugs without medical supervision. It's crucial to connect with a healthcare specialist before adopting any alternative treatments to ensure they are safe, effective, and compatible with your individual health needs and current drugs. They should be seen as complementary strategies that function in conjunction with prescribed drugs, lifestyle alterations, and regular monitoring to ensure optimal blood sugar control and general well-being

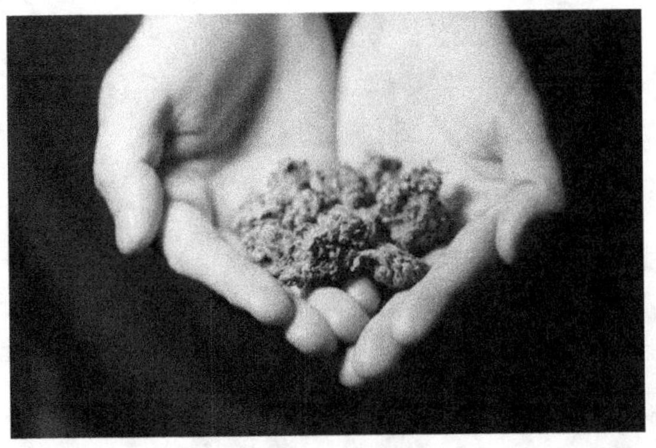

Chapter 8: Blood Sugar Control in Special Populations

Blood sugar control is essential for a range of unique populations, including pregnant women, children with diabetes, older adults, and those with specific medical conditions.

Pregnancy blood sugar control and gestational diabetes

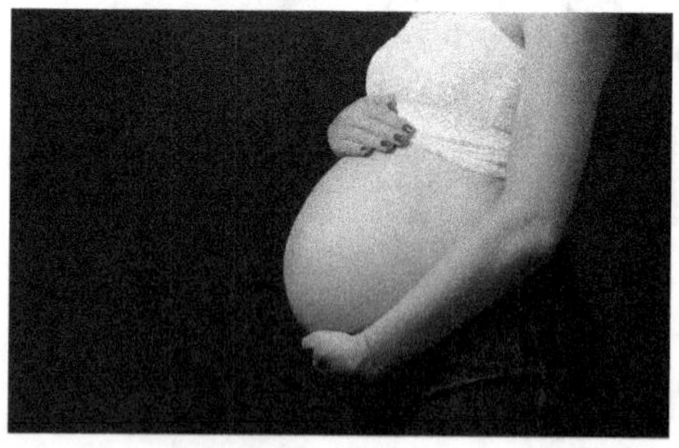

Blood sugar regulation during pregnancy is critical for both the mother's and the developing fetus's health. Gestational diabetes is one condition that demands special attention. The following is an overview of blood sugar management during pregnancy and gestational diabetes:

1. **Gestational Diabetes Screening:** Between 24 and 28 weeks of pregnancy, pregnant women are generally tested for gestational diabetes. To determine how the body processes sugar, a glucose challenge test or an oral glucose tolerance test is used. When gestational diabetes is diagnosed, blood sugar control becomes a key focus.

2. **Blood Sugar Monitoring:** Pregnant women with gestational diabetes are urged to test their blood sugar levels on a frequent basis. This includes testing blood sugar levels before and after meals for one to two hours. Blood sugar goal ranges are determined by healthcare specialists, and women are encouraged to keep track of their readings.

3. **Healthy Eating:** A well-balanced diet is vital for blood sugar regulation throughout pregnancy. Consuming a variety of

nutrient-dense foods, with a concentrate on whole grains, lean meats, fruits, vegetables, and healthy fats, is part of this. Blood sugar levels can be decreased by reducing portion sizes and spreading meals throughout the day.

4. **Physical Activity:** Regular physical activity is useful for regulating blood sugar levels during pregnancy. Low-impact exercise, like walking or swimming, can assist enhance insulin sensitivity and help maintain stable blood sugar levels. However, before beginning or modifying an exercise routine during pregnancy, talk with your doctor.

5. **Medication or Insulin Therapy:** In some circumstances, blood sugar control during pregnancy may demand the use of medication or insulin therapy. When lifestyle modifications alone are insufficient, healthcare providers may prescribe oral medicines or insulin injections to assist regulate blood sugar levels. Individual needs and regular monitoring will determine the type and dosage of medication.

6. **Regular Check-ups:** Pregnant women with gestational diabetes will have regular check-ups with healthcare specialists to monitor blood sugar levels, assess overall health, and make any required changes to the management plan. These check-ups help you to address any concerns and assure that your blood sugar levels stay within the right range.

Blood sugar control strategies for Children and teenagers

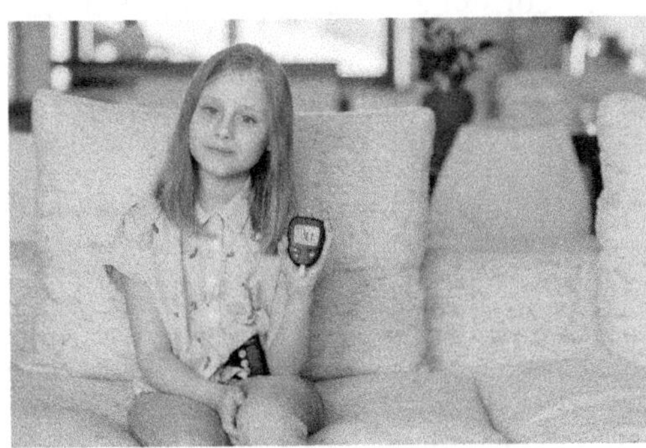

Blood sugar management in children and teens with diabetes demands a team effort from parents, carers, healthcare experts, and the kid or teenager themselves. Here are some ways to efficiently regulate blood sugar in this age group:

1. **Blood Sugar Monitoring:** Regular blood sugar monitoring is necessary to understand how the child's body responds to meals, activities, and medicine. Parents and caregivers should engage with healthcare experts to design a blood sugar monitoring regimen and target ranges. Teaching children and teenagers how to use glucose meters and involving them in blood sugar monitoring can help them take control of their health.

2. **Healthy Eating Habits:** Encourage children and teenagers to consume a well-balanced diet rich in nutrient-dense foods. Concentrate on entire grains, lean proteins, fruits and vegetables, and healthy fats. Encourage portion management and the value of frequent meals and snacks. Involve the kid or adolescent in meal preparation and planning to help them build a positive relationship with food and make healthy choices.

3. **Regular Physical Activity:** This is necessary for blood sugar regulation in children and teenagers. Encourage youngsters to participate in age-appropriate workouts or activities that they like. Physical activity enhances insulin utilization and can aid with overall blood sugar control. It is crucial to check blood sugar levels before, during, and after physical activity and to change meals or prescriptions as needed.

4. **Medication and Insulin Management**: If a child or teenager requires medication or insulin for blood sugar control, make sure they understand the value of following the prescribed schedule. Teach them how to correctly administer insulin injections or use insulin pumps, if applicable. As youngsters become more responsible for their own diabetes treatment, aid them in building drug administration routines and including them in decision-making.

5. **Diabetes Education and Support:** Provide age-appropriate diabetes and blood sugar management education to children and

teenagers. This includes learning the signs and symptoms of high and low blood sugar, knowing how to respond in emergency situations, and understanding the significance of frequent check-ups with healthcare specialists. Engage them in support groups or connect them with other diabetic peers to develop a feeling of community and shared experiences.

6. **Communication and Emotional Support:** Keep open lines of communication with children and teenagers regarding diabetes care. Encourage them to communicate their feelings, concerns, and problems associated with living with diabetes. Provide emotional support and aid them in building coping techniques for dealing with the emotional load of diabetes.

7. **School Collaboration:** Work with school staff to offer a supportive atmosphere for blood sugar management. Create a diabetes care strategy that involves monitoring blood sugar levels, delivering insulin when needed, and providing appropriate snacks or meals during the school

day. Educate teachers and school personnel on diabetes and the special needs of the child.

Blood sugar considerations for older persons and seniors

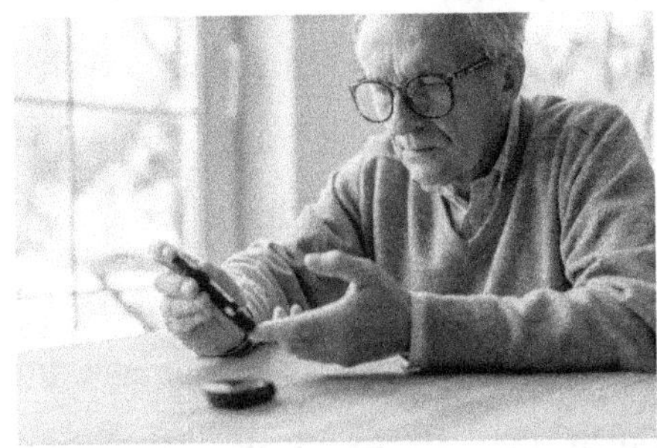 Blood sugar management is vital for older persons and seniors in order to preserve general health and avoid complications linked with diabetes or blood sugar anomalies. Here are some essential aspects to consider when managing blood sugar in this population:

1. **Regular Monitoring:** Older persons should have their blood sugar levels monitored on a regular basis to ensure they are within the target range. Regular monitoring offers essential information about how the body reacts to

nutrition, medicine, and physical activity. It also aids in the discovery of any trends or patterns that may need alterations to their management plan.

2. **Healthy Eating:** A well-balanced diet is vital for blood sugar regulation in older persons. Promote the consumption of nutrient-dense foods such as whole grains, lean meats, fruits, vegetables, and healthy fats. Portion control is crucial to avoiding carbohydrate overload, which can contribute to blood sugar rises. When designing a tailored meal plan, take into account individual nutritional needs, tastes, and any comorbidities.

3. **Medication Management:** Older persons may be taking many drugs, which may conflict with one another or impact blood sugar levels. It is vital to guarantee medication adherence and to consult with healthcare specialists to understand the potential effects on blood sugar. Adjustments or alterations to drugs may be required to ensure optimal blood sugar control.

4. **Regular Physical Activity:** Regular physical activity can help elderly persons maintain their blood sugar levels and improve their general health. Encourage them to participate in activities that are appropriate for their capacity, such as walking, swimming, or mild exercises. Before beginning or modifying an exercise program, talk with your doctor to rule out any underlying health concerns or limits.

5. **Hydration:** Older individuals should stay hydrated because it can alter blood sugar levels. Encourage them to drink plenty of water throughout the day and to avoid consuming too many sugary beverages or drinks containing artificial sweeteners.

6. **Drug Adjustments:** Age-related changes in metabolism, renal function, or liver function in older adults may impact blood sugar levels and drug responsiveness. Regular monitoring and discussion with healthcare practitioners are vital for identifying the necessity for prescription modifications or revisions.

7. **Comprehensive Healthcare Management:** Seniors should have regular check-ups with healthcare specialists to monitor blood sugar levels, review overall health, and treat any comorbid disorders. To properly manage diabetes and related health disorders, it is necessary to address any concerns, acquire adequate immunizations, and undergo required checkups.

8. **Fall Prevention:** Blood sugar abnormalities could enhance the risk of falls in the elderly. Keeping blood sugar levels steady enhances balance and reduces dizziness or weakness. Preventing falls through home safety improvements, adequate footwear, and regular exercise can help with blood sugar management indirectly.

9. **Emotional Support:** Maintaining blood sugar levels can cause emotional and psychological problems in older adults. Providing emotional support and a supportive environment may assist them in managing any stress or anxiety related to their condition.

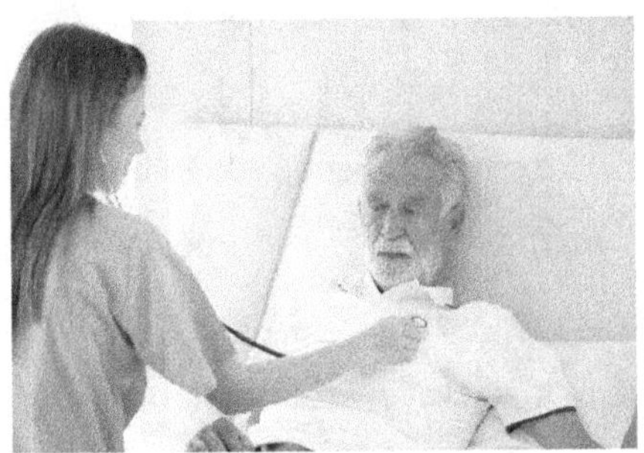

Investigating blood sugar abnormalities in persons with certain medical issues

Individuals with numerous medical diseases can have blood sugar abnormalities, and knowing these imbalances is critical for their management and overall health. Here's a quick glance at blood sugar anomalies in persons with various medical conditions:

1. **Cardiovascular Disease:** Blood sugar anomalies can occur in persons who have cardiovascular disease, such as hypertension or heart disease. High blood sugar levels can promote inflammation and blood vessel damage, raising the risk of cardiovascular complications. Controlling blood sugar levels with a healthy diet, frequent exercise, and the use of appropriate medication is crucial for cardiovascular health.

2. **Kidney Disease:** disease can alter blood sugar regulation due to diminished renal function. Because the kidneys filter and eliminate glucose, when renal function is weakened, blood sugar levels may become unstable. Close blood sugar monitoring and consultation with healthcare specialists are essential to treat renal disease and blood sugar.

3. **Liver Disease:** The liver controls blood sugar levels by storing and releasing glucose. Cirrhosis and fatty liver disease, for example, might disturb this system, resulting in blood sugar abnormalities. Blood sugar control in persons

with liver disease may involve frequent monitoring, medication adjustments, and dietary changes.

4. **Thyroid disorders:** Thyroid disorders such as hypothyroidism or hyperthyroidism, might interfere with blood sugar regulation. Hypothyroidism, or an underactive thyroid, can contribute to insulin resistance and excessive blood sugar levels. Hyperthyroidism, on the other hand, can boost insulin sensitivity and result in lower blood sugar levels. Thyroid disease care, including medication and regular monitoring, can help keep blood sugar levels stable.

5. **Pancreatic Disorders:** The pancreas is responsible for the generation of insulin, which regulates blood sugar levels. Pancreatic disorders, such as pancreatitis or pancreatic cancer, can disrupt insulin production, leading to blood sugar abnormalities. To address both the underlying pancreatic disease and blood sugar levels, constant collaboration with healthcare

experts, notably endocrinologists, and gastroenterologists, is needed.

6. **Autoimmune disorders:** Autoimmune disorders such as type 1 diabetes and celiac disease, are directly connected to blood sugar abnormalities. The immune system destroys insulin-producing cells in the pancreas in type 1 diabetes, necessitating insulin therapy for blood sugar management. Celiac disease, an autoimmune illness caused by gluten, can disturb blood sugar regulation indirectly by creating gastrointestinal difficulties that impede meal absorption.

Individuals with various medical disorders must work closely with their healthcare professionals to understand the specific impact on blood sugar regulation and build tailored management programs. This may require regular blood sugar monitoring, proper medication or insulin therapy, dietary adjustments, and lifestyle changes. Individuals can enhance their general health and well-being by addressing both the underlying medical disease and blood sugar abnormalities.

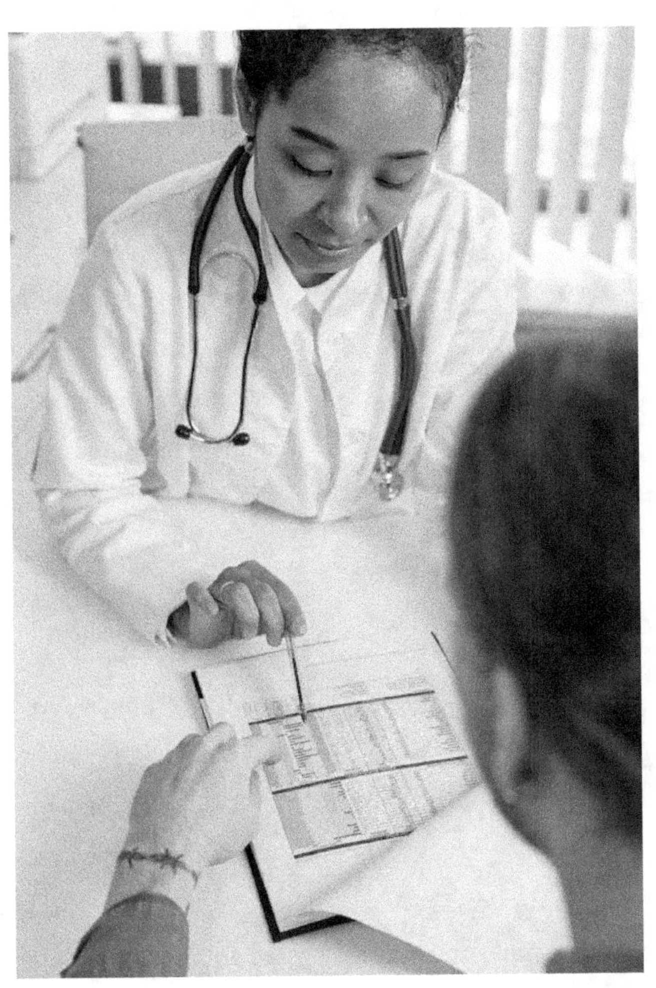

Chapter 9: Blood Sugar Monitoring and Tracking

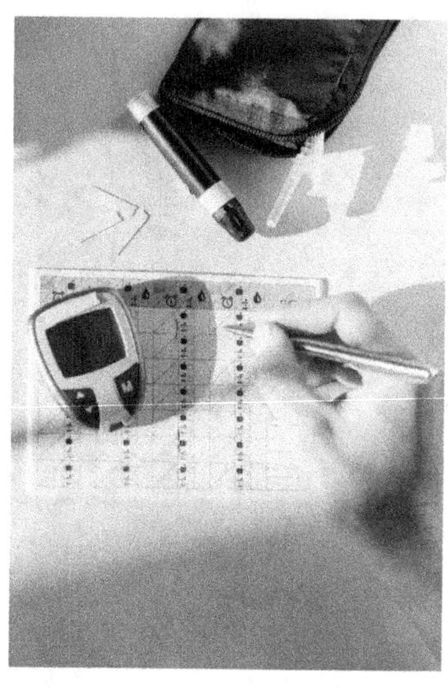

Blood sugar monitoring and tracking are essential components of managing blood sugar levels successfully. Regular monitoring delivers crucial information on how the body responds to a multitude of factors, including nutrition, physical exercise, drugs, and stress. When it comes to blood sugar monitoring and tracking, keep the following aspects in mind:

1. **Importance of Monitoring:** is vital because it allows people to understand their current blood

sugar situation and make informed health decisions. It aids in the identification of patterns, trends, and potential imbalances that may demand alterations to their diabetic care regimen.

2. **Methods of Monitoring:** Fingerstick blood glucose meters, continuous glucose monitoring (CGM) devices, and flash glucose monitoring systems can all be used to monitor blood sugar levels. Individual preferences, lifestyle, and healthcare practitioner recommendations all have an impact on the technique employed.

3. **Monitoring Frequency:** The frequency of blood sugar monitoring varies depending on the type and severity of diabetes, treatment approach, and individual needs. It could be multiple times per day or once a week. Healthcare professionals advise patients on the proper monitoring plan for them.

4. **Target Blood Sugar Ranges:** Target blood sugar ranges are commonly determined by healthcare practitioners based on criteria such as age, overall health, and specific diabetes

treatment goals. Individuals might employ monitoring to discover if their blood sugar levels are normal or if they need to make improvements.

5. **Tracking Tools:** A range of tools and apps are available to track and analyze blood sugar levels over time. These technologies assist users in spotting patterns, trends, and potential triggers for blood sugar fluctuations, leading to improved diabetes therapy.

6. **Communication with Healthcare Professionals:** Sharing blood sugar data with healthcare specialists at routine check-ups or virtual visits enables a thorough examination of trends and, if necessary, adjustments to the diabetes management plan.

7. **Self-Reflection and Decision Making:** Tracking and monitoring blood sugar levels encourage patients to become more involved in their diabetes treatment. Individuals can make more informed decisions about diet, exercise, medicine, and lifestyle behaviors if they

understand how various things affect their blood sugar.

The value of maintaining a blood sugar diary and tracking trends over time

Maintaining a blood sugar record and tracking patterns over time is crucial for effective diabetes control. Here are some essential components that underscore the need of keeping a blood sugar log:

1. **Progress Monitoring:** A blood sugar log retains an accurate record of blood sugar levels over time. By checking their blood sugar levels on a daily basis, people may examine their progress, uncover patterns, and assess how well their present management plan is working.

2. **Identifying Triggers and Patterns:** By keeping a blood sugar record, patients can notice blood sugar triggers such as certain foods, medications, physical exercise, or stress. People

can keep their blood sugar levels constant by detecting patterns and making appropriate alterations to their lifestyle, medicine, or diet choices.

3. **Collaboration with Medical Professionals:** Sharing blood sugar log data with medical professionals during check-ups or consultations allows them to look for patterns and make informed treatment decisions. It helps healthcare providers to alter counsel based on a more thorough assessment of the effectiveness of present management methods.

4. **Making Informed Decisions:** A blood sugar log empowers individuals to make informed decisions about their diabetes management. By understanding how specific factors impact their blood sugar levels, individuals can modify their meal plans, adjust medication doses, or incorporate more physical activity to achieve better blood sugar control.

5. **Early Detection of Problems:** Regularly tracking blood sugar levels helps individuals identify any potential problems or abnormalities

at an early stage. It enables them to seek medical attention promptly if blood sugar levels consistently fall outside the target range, reducing the risk of complications associated with uncontrolled blood sugar levels.

6. **Motivation and Accountability:** Maintaining a blood sugar log can serve as a source of motivation and accountability. Seeing improvements and stable blood sugar trends can provide encouragement to continue practicing healthy habits. It also highlights the impact of certain lifestyle choices on blood sugar, reinforcing the importance of adherence to the management plan.

7. **Effective Communication:** A blood sugar log facilitates effective communication between individuals and their healthcare team. Sharing the log during appointments allows for meaningful discussions, enables healthcare professionals to provide targeted advice, and fosters a collaborative approach to diabetes management.

By consistently keeping a blood sugar log and tracking trends over time, individuals gain valuable insights into their diabetes management. It empowers them to take an active role in their health, make informed decisions, and work closely with healthcare professionals to optimize blood sugar control and overall well-being.

Interpreting blood sugar readings and making adjustments to lifestyle or medication

Interpreting blood sugar readings is an essential skill for individuals managing diabetes. Understanding how to analyze these readings and make appropriate adjustments to lifestyle or medication can help maintain optimal blood sugar control. Here are some steps to consider:

1. **Know the Target Range:** It is important to be familiar with the target blood sugar range recommended by healthcare professionals. This range may vary depending on factors such as

age, overall health, and specific diabetes management goals. Typically, a target range for fasting blood sugar is between 80-130 mg/dL (4.4-7.2 mmol/L), and 2 hours after meals, it should be less than 180 mg/dL (10.0 mmol/L).

2. **Monitor Trends:** Look for patterns and trends in blood sugar readings over time. Keep a record of blood sugar levels in a log or use digital tracking tools to visualize trends. Identifying consistent high or low readings and understanding when they occur can help pinpoint potential triggers.

3. **Identify Potential Triggers:** Consider factors that may contribute to blood sugar fluctuations, such as food choices, physical activity, medication adherence, stress levels, illness, or changes in routine. By analyzing the circumstances surrounding abnormal blood sugar readings, you can determine potential triggers and make informed adjustments.

4. **Lifestyle Adjustments:** Lifestyle modifications play a significant role in blood sugar management. Based on blood sugar readings and

identified patterns, consider making adjustments to your diet, exercise routine, stress management techniques, and sleep habits. For example, if consistently high blood sugar levels occur after meals, you may need to reassess your carbohydrate intake or portion sizes.

5. **Medication Adjustments:** If lifestyle changes alone do not achieve the desired blood sugar control, medication adjustments may be necessary. Consult with your healthcare professional before making any changes to your medication regimen. They can assess your blood sugar log, review trends, and determine if medication adjustments, such as dose changes or timing modifications, are appropriate.

6. **Regular Communication with Healthcare Professionals:** It is essential to maintain regular communication with your healthcare team. Share your blood sugar log during appointments or consultations, and discuss any concerns or challenges you are facing. Collaborate with them to make informed decisions about lifestyle

adjustments or medication changes based on blood sugar readings and patterns.

7. **Continuous Monitoring:** Regularly monitor your blood sugar levels to assess the impact of lifestyle and medication adjustments. By tracking and evaluating the effectiveness of the changes made, you can determine if further adjustments are necessary or if the current approach is achieving the desired blood sugar control.

The Role of continuous glucose monitoring (CGM) Devices and their benefits

Continuous glucose monitoring (CGM) devices play a vital role in diabetes management by providing real-time information about blood sugar levels throughout the day and night. These devices offer several benefits that enhance blood sugar control and improve overall quality of life. Here's an overview of the role of CGM devices and their benefits:

1. **Real-Time Blood Sugar Data:** CGM devices continuously measure glucose levels in the interstitial fluid, providing real-time data on blood sugar trends, highs, and lows. This information helps individuals make immediate and informed decisions about their diabetes management, allowing for timely interventions.

2. **Early Detection of Trends and Patterns:** CGM devices detect trends and patterns in blood sugar levels over time. They provide detailed insights into how food choices, physical activity, stress, medication, and other factors impact blood sugar. By identifying patterns, individuals can proactively address issues and make targeted adjustments to their lifestyle or medication to maintain stable blood sugar levels.

3. **Hypoglycemia and Hyperglycemia Alerts:** CGM devices can be set to deliver alerts when blood sugar levels fall too low (hypoglycemia) or rise too high (hyperglycemia). These alerts

serve as valuable reminders, particularly during sleep or times when individuals may not be aware of their blood sugar fluctuations. Prompt notifications allow for timely intervention and can help prevent severe episodes.

4. **Reduced Fingerstick Testing:** CGM devices minimize the need for frequent fingerstick testing, providing a more convenient and comfortable monitoring experience. While fingerstick testing is still necessary for calibration and confirming blood sugar readings, CGM systems significantly reduce the number of required fingerstick tests.

5. **Data Visualization and Analysis:** CGM systems come with easy-to-use software or smartphone apps that display blood sugar data in graphs, charts, and trend reports. These visualizations aid users and healthcare professionals in evaluating data more thoroughly, recognizing patterns, and altering management plans accordingly.

6. **Improved Quality of Life:** CGM devices allow users more flexibility and peace of mind. They

can participate in activities like exercise or vacation with confidence because their blood sugar levels are constantly monitored. CGM systems lessen the stress of frequent blood sugar measurement, allowing users to focus more on their daily activities and live healthier lives.

7. **Enhanced Diabetes Management:** Diabetes management is enhanced because CGM devices enable a more proactive and tailored approach to diabetes control. CGM systems enable users to make informed decisions about their food, exercise, medicine, and lifestyle by delivering real-time data, insights into patterns, and warnings for highs and lows. This proactive approach to diabetes therapy may result in better blood sugar control and a lower risk of diabetes-related complications.

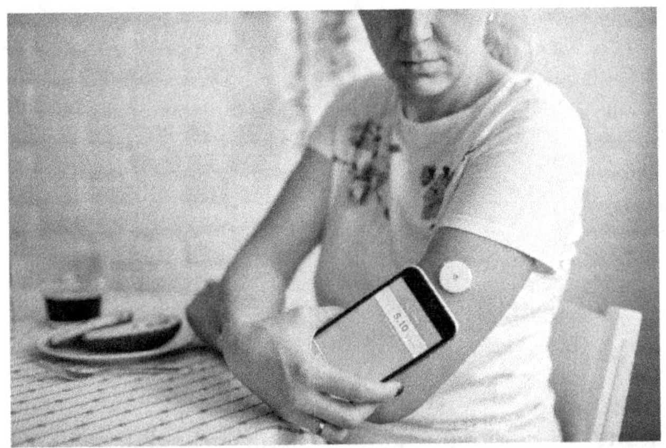

CGM devices should be utilized in coordination with healthcare experts. They can advise on device selection, data interpretation, and modifications to the diabetic care plan based on CGM readings. CGM devices are a great tool that can drastically enhance diabetes management and overall well-being by supplementing traditional blood sugar monitoring methods.

Chapter 10: Long–Term Blood Sugar Balance and Prevention

Long-term blood sugar control is critical for diabetes patients to avoid problems and maintain general health. Individuals can successfully manage their blood sugar levels and limit the possibility of long-term issues by employing proactive techniques. Here's a full discussion of long-term blood sugar regulation and prevention:

1. **Diabetes knowledge:** Long-term blood sugar balance requires knowledge. Individuals should seek comprehensive diabetes education programs to obtain a better awareness of the ailment, its treatment, and the requirement for blood sugar management. Individuals benefit from education when making educated

decisions, adhering to treatment regimens, and managing their health proactively.

2. **Healthy Eating:** A balanced and healthy diet has a vital function in long-term blood sugar homeostasis. Consume a variety of substantial meals that include vegetables, fruits, whole grains, lean meats, and healthy fats. Control portion sizes, practice carbohydrate counting, and avoid processed foods, sugary beverages, and high-glycemic-index items. For professional food planning, visit a licensed nutritionist.

3. **Regular Physical Activity:** Maintaining long-term blood sugar homeostasis demands regular physical activity. Exercise enhances insulin sensitivity, aids in weight management, and reduces blood sugar levels. Aim for at least 150 minutes per week of moderate-intensity aerobic activity, as well as strength training activities. Before beginning any new workout plan, talk with a healthcare professional.

4. **Medication Adherence:** Maintaining long-term blood sugar homeostasis needs continuous and correct administration of prescription

medications. Follow prescription directions exactly as given by your healthcare practitioner and consult with them before making any modifications. Adherence to drug regimens allows for improved blood sugar management and lowers the risk of problems.

5. **Regular Blood Sugar Monitoring:** Regular blood sugar monitoring offers vital information for blood sugar control and aids in the detection of trends and patterns. Monitor blood sugar levels as recommended by healthcare specialists, and keep a diary to document progress and make any modifications. Regular monitoring helps individuals to take proactive efforts to maintain long-term blood sugar homeostasis.

6. **Stress Management:** Chronic stress may have a detrimental impact on blood sugar levels. Implement stress-reduction tactics such as relaxation exercises, mindfulness, deep breathing, and engaging in calm-promoting activities. Adequate sleep, social support, and indulging in hobbies can all benefit from stress reduction.

7. **Check-ups with Healthcare Professionals:** Regular check-ups with healthcare professionals are crucial for long-term blood sugar management. Healthcare specialists can monitor overall health, analyze blood sugar logs, alter treatment programs as needed, and provide guidance on how to avoid issues. Attend suggested screenings for eye, kidney, and nerve health to detect and address potential problems early.

8. **Tobacco and alcohol management:** Smoking and excessive drinking can complicate blood sugar control and raise the risk of complications. Quit smoking and minimize alcohol use to moderate levels, or avoid it completely, as prescribed by healthcare professionals.

9. **Maintaining a healthy weight:** This is crucial for long-term blood sugar regulation. Aim for a healthy BMI (body mass index) range and seek individualized weight control solutions from healthcare specialists or trained dietitians.

10. **Support systems:** Building a support system, which includes family, friends, and diabetic

support groups, can provide emotional and practical help for long-term blood sugar control. Connecting with individuals who have had similar experiences can be empowering and aid in motivation.

Individuals can accomplish long-term blood sugar regulation and avoid diabetic complications by employing these comprehensive measures. It is vital to engage closely with healthcare providers to build a personalized management plan that fits individual requirements and goals.

Maintaining blood sugar balance following initial improvements

After initial improvements, maintaining blood sugar balance is critical for long-term health and diabetes treatment. Following favorable changes and initial breakthroughs in blood sugar control, it is vital to maintain healthy behaviors and remain watchful. Here are some crucial considerations for maintaining blood sugar balance:

1. **Consistency:** This is crucial when it comes to maintaining blood sugar equilibrium. Maintain your diabetes treatment plan, which includes a nutritious diet, frequent physical activity, medication adherence, and regular blood sugar monitoring. Avoid relapsing to prior behaviors and retain the remarkable achievements you've gained.

2. **Ongoing Education:** Stay up to date on the most recent diabetes research and developments. Continue to educate yourself through trustworthy sources, attend diabetes education programs, and stay in touch with healthcare professionals for help and support.

3. **Self-Monitoring:** As indicated by your healthcare practitioner, continue to test your blood sugar levels on a regular basis. Tracking your blood sugar levels and observing trends

will assist you in spotting any potential concerns or patterns that require correction.

4. **Regular Health Check-ups:** Maintain regular check-ups with your healthcare specialists to analyze your overall health and reassess your diabetes treatment plan. They can analyze your progress, make any required adjustments, and provide direction to assist you in maintaining your blood sugar balance.

5. **Stress Management:** Because persistent stress can alter blood sugar levels, it is vital to handle stress efficiently. Incorporate stress-reduction tactics such as relaxation exercises, mindfulness, hobbies, and seeking social support. Adequate sleep and self-care routines can help with stress management.

6. **Lifestyle Changes:** Maintain healthy lifestyle choices that increase blood sugar homeostasis. Adopting a balanced diet, engaging in regular physical activity, getting enough sleep, managing weight, and avoiding tobacco and excessive alcohol intake are all part of this.

7. **Support Network:** Surround yourself with family, friends, or support groups who understand your path and can offer encouragement and accountability. Sharing your struggles and experiences with others can be uplifting and encouraging.

8. **Adjustments as Needed:** Be willing to make modifications to your diabetes control plan as necessary. Your healthcare providers may vary your medication, food, or exercise regimes based on your changing needs and any changes in your health status.

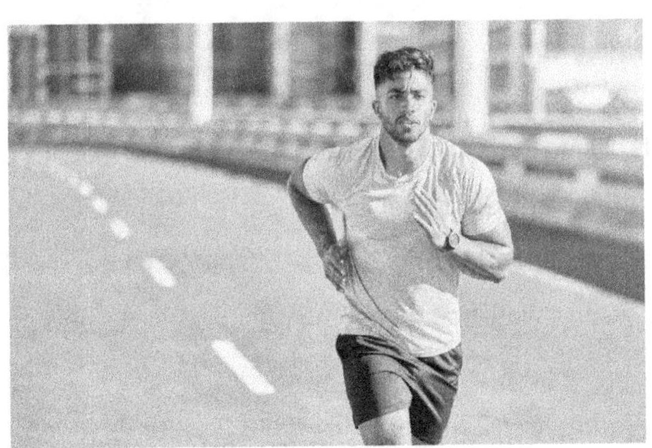

Conclusion

"Glucose Revolution Code" is not just a book; it's a game-changer, a path to a happier and more fulfilling life. By going into the pages of this exceptional guide, you will obtain a comprehensive understanding of your body, your blood sugar, and the intricate relationship between the two. With its wealth of knowledge, empowering strategies, and scrumptious recipes, the book becomes a trusted companion on your journey towards balanced blood sugar levels.

No longer will you feel at the mercy of sugar spikes or energy crashes. Instead, armed with the wisdom and tools found within the Glucose Revolution Code, you'll regain control over your health and vitality. This book is your key to unlocking a new chapter, where stability, clarity, and well-being become the norm.

The time to take charge of your health is now. Say goodbye to the pitfalls of unstable blood sugar and embrace a future of optimal wellness. Let the Glucose

Revolution Code be your guide as you embark on a transformative adventure towards a vibrant and fulfilling life. Your journey for balanced blood sugar starts here. Empower yourself, live your health, and live your best life.

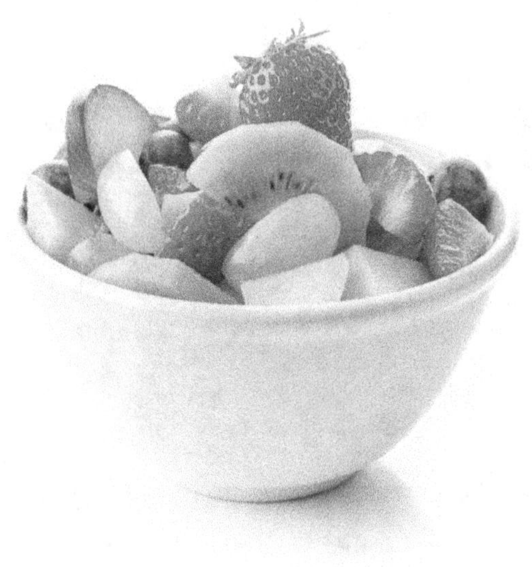

Inspirational success stories and testimonials from people who have achieved long-term blood sugar balance

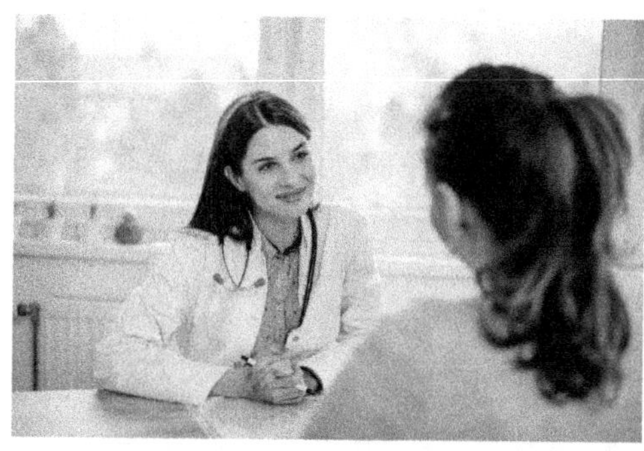

Success stories and testimonies from people who have obtained long-term blood sugar balance can be immensely encouraging and give hope to those who are on a similar journey. Here are a handful of such examples:

1. **Sarah's Story:** Sarah was diagnosed with type 2 diabetes and struggled for years to maintain her

blood sugar levels normal. She was able to lose weight and improve her blood sugar management by making lifestyle adjustments such as eating a balanced diet and exercising frequently. Sarah is no longer on medicine and lives an active, healthy lifestyle.

2. **Mark's Story:** During his wife's pregnancy, Mark was diagnosed with gestational diabetes. He embraced a balanced diet and regular physical activity to promote his family's health. His attention to blood sugar regulation benefited not just his wife during her pregnancy but also contributed to long-term benefits in his own health. Mark continues to put his health first and serves as a role model for his children.

3. **Emily's Story:** Emily was diagnosed with type 1 diabetes at a young age. Despite the hurdles, she never let her illness hold her back. Emily has succeeded thanks to meticulous self-care, such as blood sugar monitoring, insulin management, and good lifestyle choices. She has run marathons, climbed mountains, and inspired people with her power and perseverance.

4. **Joshua's Lifestyle Change:** After being diagnosed with prediabetes, Joshua acknowledged the need of making lifestyle changes to avoid the progression to type 2 diabetes. He made considerable dietary modifications, including more healthy foods and limiting his intake of sugary beverages and processed snacks. Joshua was able to rectify his prediabetes and maintain stable blood sugar levels with the aid of his healthcare team and a devoted mindset.

These success stories indicate that long-term blood sugar balance is feasible with work, education, support, and a dedication to healthy practices. Each person's journey is unique, but these examples highlight the importance of making healthy choices and taking ownership of one's health.

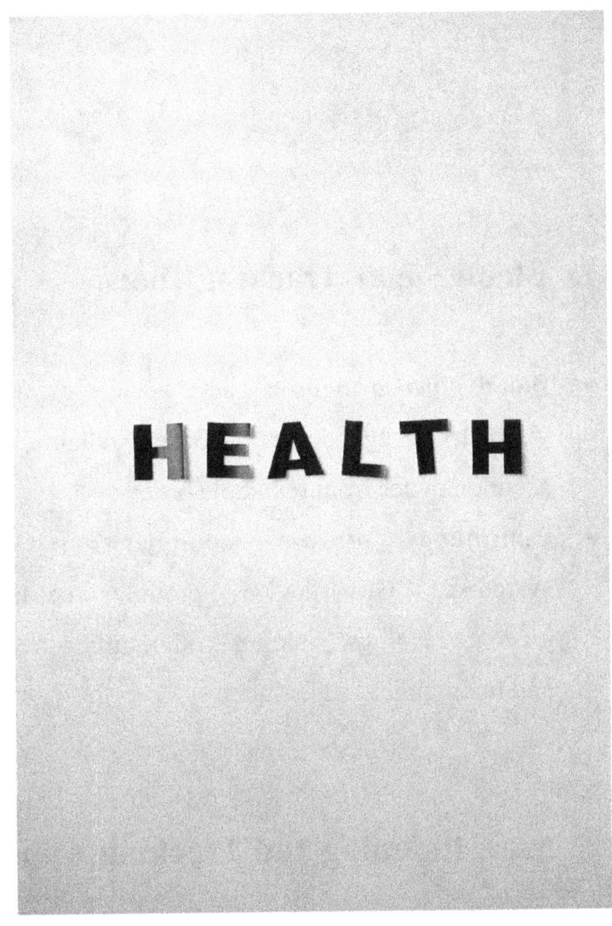
HEALTH

Appendix: Resources and Tools

1. Blood Sugar Tracking Tools:

- **Blood glucose meters:** These devices measure your blood sugar levels. Choose a reliable and accurate meter from reputable brands.
- **Continuous glucose monitoring (CGM) systems:** CGM devices provide real-time glucose readings, helping you monitor trends and make timely adjustments.

2. Meal Planning and Tracking Apps:

- **MyFitnessPal:** This popular app allows you to track your meals, log your food intake, and monitor macronutrients, including carbohydrates, proteins, and fats.

- **Carbohydrate Counting Apps:** Apps like "Carb Manager" or "MyNetDiary" help you estimate and track carbohydrate intake, aiding in blood sugar management.

3. Diabetes Education and Support Programs:

- **American Diabetes Association (ADA):** Visit the ADA website for educational resources, diabetes management guidelines, and information on local support groups.
- **Diabetes Online Communities:** Engage with online communities such as Diabetes Daily, TuDiabetes, or Reddit's r/diabetes to connect with others facing similar challenges and share experiences.

4. Exercise and Fitness Resources:

- **Fitbit or Other Fitness Trackers:** Use a fitness tracker to monitor your physical activity, set goals, and track progress.

- **Exercise Apps:** Explore exercise apps like Nike Training Club, MyFitnessPal, or Fitbod for guided workouts, exercise plans, and tracking features.

5. Health and Wellness Apps:

- **Headspace:** This mindfulness and meditation app can help with stress management and relaxation techniques.

- **Sleep Cycle:** Monitor and improve your sleep quality using sleep tracking apps like Sleep Cycle, which analyzes your sleep patterns and wakes you up at the optimal time.

6. Healthcare Professionals:

- **Registered Dietitians:** Consult with a registered dietitian who specializes in diabetes and blood sugar management for personalized meal planning and guidance.

- **Certified Diabetes Educators (CDE):** CDEs provide education and support for individuals managing diabetes, helping with medication management, lifestyle changes, and blood sugar monitoring.

Glossary of key terms related to blood sugar and diabetes

Here is a glossary of key terms related to blood sugar and diabetes:

1. **Blood Sugar:** The concentration of glucose (sugar) in the blood. It is also known as blood glucose level.

2. **Insulin:** A hormone produced by the pancreas that regulates blood sugar levels by allowing glucose to enter cells for energy. In diabetes, there is either insufficient insulin production (type 1 diabetes) or ineffective use of insulin (type 2 diabetes).

3. **Glucose:** A simple sugar that serves as the primary source of energy for the body's cells. It is derived from the breakdown of carbohydrates in the diet.

4. **Hyperglycemia:** High blood sugar levels, typically defined as blood glucose levels above the normal range. It is a common symptom of uncontrolled diabetes.

5. **Hypoglycemia:** Low blood sugar levels, typically defined as blood glucose levels below the normal range. It can occur in individuals with diabetes who take insulin or certain medications.

6. **Glycemic Index (GI):** A ranking system that measures how carbohydrates in food affect blood sugar levels. Foods with a high GI raise blood sugar levels more quickly than foods with a low GI.

7. **Glycemic Load (GL):** A measure that takes into account both the quality (GI) and quantity of carbohydrates in food. It provides a more accurate assessment of the impact of food on blood sugar levels.

8. **A1C:** Also known as glycated hemoglobin, it is a blood test that measures the average blood sugar levels over the past 2-3 months. It is

commonly used to diagnose and monitor diabetes.

9. **Prediabetes:** A condition in which blood sugar levels are higher than normal but not high enough to be diagnosed as diabetes. It is a warning sign of increased risk for developing type 2 diabetes.

10. **Ketones:** Chemical substances produced when the body breaks down fat for energy in the absence of sufficient insulin. High levels of ketones can occur in individuals with uncontrolled diabetes, leading to a condition called diabetic ketoacidosis.

11. **Pancreas:** A gland located behind the stomach that produces insulin and other hormones necessary for digestion and blood sugar regulation.

12. **Diabetes Mellitus:** A chronic metabolic disorder characterized by elevated blood sugar levels due to either insufficient insulin production (type 1 diabetes) or ineffective use of insulin (type 2 diabetes).

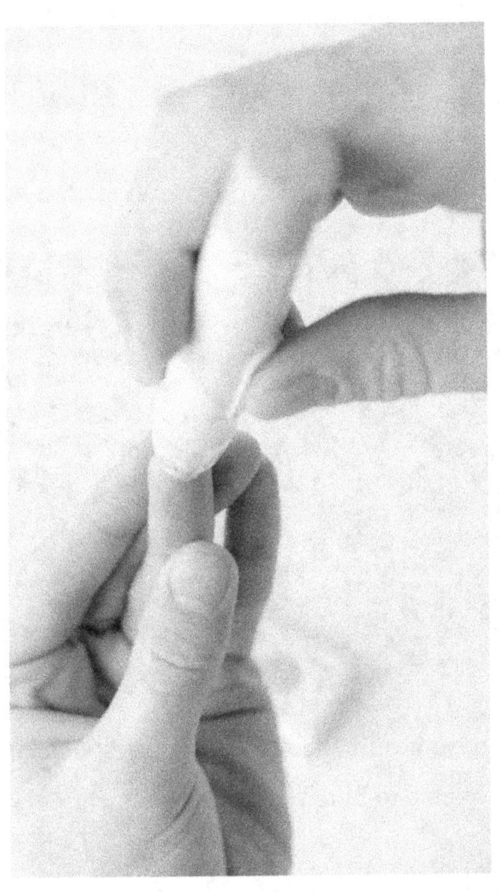

Frequently asked questions and their answers related to blood sugar management

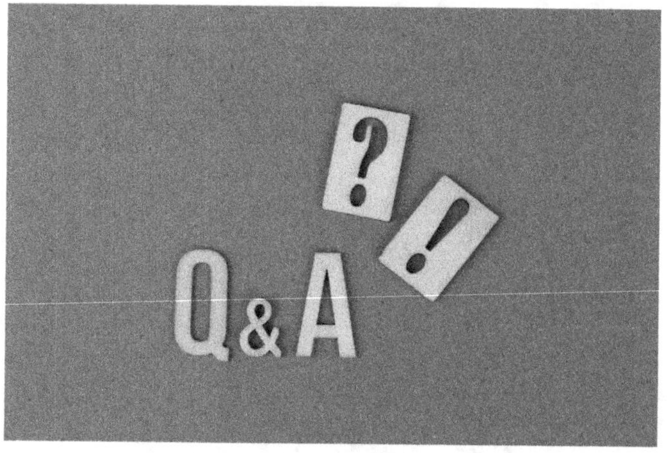

Here are some frequently asked questions and their answers related to blood sugar management:

Q: What is considered a normal blood sugar range?

A: A normal fasting blood sugar level is typically between 70-99 mg/dL (3.9-5.5 mmol/L). Postprandial (after eating) blood sugar levels should generally be below 140 mg/dL (7.8 mmol/L) after two hours.

Q: How often should I check my blood sugar levels?

A: The frequency of blood sugar monitoring may vary depending on individual circumstances and the advice of your healthcare provider. In general, individuals with type 1 diabetes may need to monitor their blood sugar multiple times a day, while those with type 2 diabetes may check it as recommended by their healthcare team.

Q: What lifestyle changes can help manage blood sugar levels?

A: Lifestyle changes that can help manage blood sugar levels include adopting a balanced diet, engaging in regular physical activity, maintaining a healthy weight, managing stress levels, getting adequate sleep, and avoiding tobacco and excessive alcohol consumption.

Q: Can exercise help lower blood sugar levels?

A: Yes, exercise can help lower blood sugar levels by increasing insulin sensitivity and promoting glucose uptake by muscles. It is important to consult with your healthcare provider to determine the appropriate exercise routine and any precautions needed.

Q: Can certain foods help stabilize blood sugar levels?

A: Yes, certain foods can help stabilize blood sugar levels. Focus on consuming a balanced diet that includes whole grains, lean proteins, healthy fats, and plenty of fruits and vegetables. Limiting processed foods, sugary drinks, and foods high in refined carbohydrates is also beneficial.

Q: Can stress affect blood sugar levels?

A: Yes, stress can affect blood sugar levels. During periods of stress, the body releases stress hormones that can cause an increase in blood sugar levels. Managing stress through relaxation techniques, exercise, and healthy coping strategies can help maintain stable blood sugar levels.

Q: What are the warning signs of high or low blood sugar?

A: The warning signs of high blood sugar (hyperglycemia) may include increased thirst, frequent urination, fatigue, blurred vision, and slow wound healing. The warning signs of low blood sugar (hypoglycemia) may include shakiness, dizziness, confusion, sweating, and rapid heartbeat.

Q: How can I prevent complications associated with uncontrolled blood sugar levels?

A: To prevent complications, it is essential to maintain stable blood sugar levels through a combination of medication, lifestyle changes, and regular medical check-ups. Adhering to a blood sugar management plan, taking prescribed medications, and staying proactive in your healthcare are key steps in preventing complications.

BLOOD SUGAR TRACKER

Date	Time	Blood Sugar Level
1		
2		
3		
4		
5		

6		
7		
8		
9		
10		
11		

12		
13		
14		
15		

16		
17		
18		
19		
20		
21		

22		
23		
24		
25		
26		
27		

28		
29		
30		

A simple spreadsheet to record your blood sugar readings, including date, time (fasting and/or post-meals) and corresponding glucose levels.